Resource CD-ROM

for

Hands Heal Essentials

Documentation for Massage Therapists

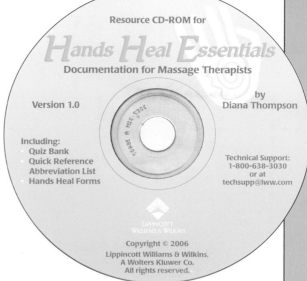

Resource CD-ROM for

Hands Heal Essentials
Documentation for Massage Therapists

Version 1.0

by
Diana Thompson

Including:
- Quiz Bank
- Quick Reference
Abbreviation List
- Hands Heal Forms

Technical Support:
1-800-638-3030
or at
techsupp@lww.com

LIPPINCOTT
WILLIAMS & WILKINS

Copyright © 2006
Lippincott Williams & Wilkins,
A Wolters Kluwer Co.
All rights reserved.

As a bonus for you, Lippincott Williams & Wilkins has included an interactive CD-ROM with tools to enhance your learning and your practice!

This resource is the perfect tool to help you prepare for exams, to reinforce what you have learned, and to make your paperwork easier.

The CD-ROM includes:

- A quiz tool with approximately 150 multiple-choice questions so you can test your knowledge and study for tests. Choose study mode or test mode, and even e-mail your results to your instructor. A comprehensive exam is offered and rationales are given so you can understand the reasoning behind the correct answer.

- The blank forms from the book that you can print out and use and practice.

- Quick-reference list including symbols and abbreviations commonly used in documentation.

For technical support, contact 1-800-638-3030 or techsupp@lww.com.

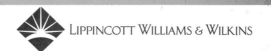

LIPPINCOTT WILLIAMS & WILKINS

HANDS HEAL ESSENTIALS:

Documentation for Massage Therapists

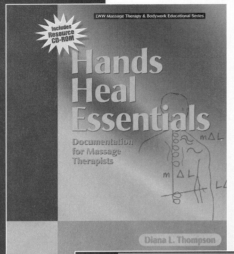
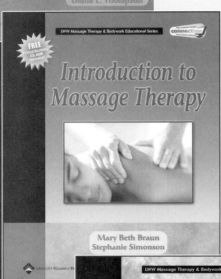
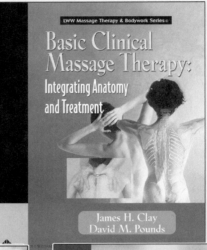
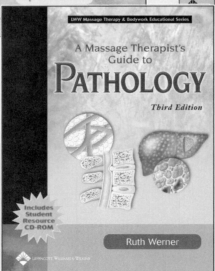
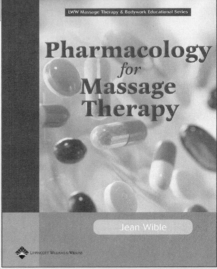
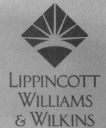

Hands Heal Essentials

Documentation for Massage Therapists

Diana L. Thompson

Licensed Massage Practitioner
Seattle, Washington

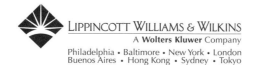

LIPPINCOTT WILLIAMS & WILKINS
A **Wolters Kluwer** Company

Philadelphia • Baltimore • New York • London
Buenos Aires • Hong Kong • Sydney • Tokyo

Executive Editor: Peter J. Darcy
Managing Editor: Anne Seitz, Hearthside Publishing Services
Editorial Coordinator: Katherine Staples
Marketing Manager: Christen Murphy
Associate Production Manager: Kevin P. Johnson
Designer: Risa Clow
Compositor: Schawk, Inc.; Publishing Solutions for Retail, Book, and Catalog
Printer: Courier—Westford

Lippincott Williams & Wilkins
530 Walnut Street
Philadelphia, PA 19106–3621 USA

Printed in the United States of America

Library of Congress Cataloging-in-Publication Data

Thompson, Diana L.
  Hands heal essentials: documentation for massage therapists / Diana L. Thompson.—1st ed.
    p. cm.
  Includes index.
   ISBN 0-7817-5758-4 (alk. paper)
  1. Massage theraphy—Practice I. Title.
RM722. T483 2005
615.8'22—dc22

2005008568

To purchase additional copies of this book, call our customer service department at **(800) 638-3030** or fax orders to **(301) 824-7390.** International customers should call **(301) 714-2324.**

Visit Lippincott Williams & Wilkins on the Internet: http://www.LWW.com. Lippincott Williams & Wilkins customer service representatives are available from 8:30 am to 6:00 pm, EST.

05 06 07 08
1 2 3 4 5 6 7 8 9 10

I dedicate this edition to Kenai: Your positive attitude and playful sweetness are an inspiration. "Thank you God for my perfect health." I hope to share in your next life!

Preface

Background of Hands Heal Essentials

Hands Heal Essentials began as a longer book titled *Hands Heal*, which was conceived in the early 1990s. At that time, complementary and alternative medicine was receiving a lot of press and catching the attention of mainstream health care systems. Massage therapists, bodyworkers, movement therapists, and energy workers were receiving client referrals from physicians, many for the first time. Increasingly, manual therapy services were being covered by insurance plans and massage therapists were being licensed as health care providers.

Not everyone in allopathic medicine greeted the complementary providers with open arms. Skepticism was widespread. Many questioned the validity of manual therapies. Insurance carriers demanded statistics and scientific studies proving that treatment was curative and not palliative. Few were found. Independent medical examinations were implemented early in personal injury cases, and health insurance utilization review boards audited practitioners, in attempts to deny or to limit the use of manual therapies.

In this atmosphere of litigation and peer reviews, charting focused on proving the legitimacy of the practitioners and their modalities. I wrote the first edition of *Hands Heal* to prepare massage therapists for the charting requirements of those skeptical times. My information was based on years of experience in the early stages of the integration of massage therapy into health care. My teachers were chiropractors, attorneys, and insurance adjusters. I had been videotaped for depositions, had given testimony in court, had submitted narratives to lawyers, and had seen my charts reviewed by utilization management panels. On the upside, when my claims were denied, the decisions were reversed after I submitted convincing progress reports. Also, I filed liens in county courthouses and had requested letters of guarantee from attorneys, and, as a result, I received payment in full when others were being asked to cut their bills in half. I wanted to share what I had learned.

Much has changed in a short time. Massage therapy is now considered a viable treatment option for many people and is a covered benefit in an increasing number of insurance plans across the United States. Because of this widespread integration of manual therapies into private health care benefit packages, charting requirements have also changed. The focus of documentation continues to shift from legitimizing the practitioners and validating massage techniques to proving that the treatments improve client outcomes and cost less than traditional treatments. The shift demands progress-oriented functional outcomes reporting, a style of charting adopted recently by physical therapists and other health care providers. Progress becomes apparent when the client's quality of life improves. Quality of life is measured through functional outcomes—the client's increased ability to participate in activities of daily life.

Current research supports the emphasis on functional outcomes. A randomized trial studying the effects of various alternative therapies in treating persistent low back pain was conducted at the Center for Health Studies in Washington State. Dan Cherkin, PhD, Senior Scientific Investigator, concluded that therapeutic massage is an effective treatment for persistent low back pain because massage significantly improves the client's ability to function (such as in the ability to walk up stairs and put on socks). There was not a statistically significant reduction in symptoms, though there was a correlation between massage and the reduction of medication (Cherkin D, Eisenberg D, Street J, et al. Randomized trial comparing traditional Chinese medical acupuncture, therapeutic massage, and self-care education for chronic low back pain. Arch Intern Med 2001;161).

When we, as massage therapists, persist in trying to demonstrate client progress through a reduction in symptoms, we are less able to provide our clients with encouraging results or to prove the curative nature of our modalities. When we demonstrate client progress through improved function, however, we will validate manual modalities successfully.

This shift in charting is exciting. Practitioners and clients alike enjoy the focus on improving function. Setting functional goals and charting functional outcomes engages clients in their healing, inviting them to participate in all levels of healing. Functional outcomes reporting fits into a SOAP format with few adjustments, and the second and third editions of *Hands Heal* make the transition to functional outcomes reporting easy.

The Creation of Hands Heal Essentials

Although much of the massage therapy profession is wading into the medical waters, many therapists are choosing to work within the wellness paradigm. On-site massage is on the rise in the workplace, day spas are popping up in suburban neighborhoods, and sports venues are no longer complete without massage therapists at the finish line.

Standard medical documentation is excessive in these venues. But because of the inclusion of massage therapy into the medical arena, massage therapists are held accountable as health care providers. Recordkeeping is expected by other members of the health care team and by our clients who use massage therapy to stay healthy and active.

Hands Heal Essentials is devoted to the hows and whys of charting wellness sessions. Massage therapy enhances wellness in addition to treating health conditions. Regardless of its intent, massage therapy is a health care service and therefore must be documented. However, extensive documentation using the SOAP format is not necessary in wellness care. Instead, this *Essentials* edition offers abbreviated intake forms and brief wellness charts for recording the client information essential to providing safe and skillful massage therapy—and removes references to injury treatment and insurance billing, which are covered in detail in *Hands Heal*.

SOAP charting is included in *Hands Heal Essentials* for those who cross over into treatment massage but are not yet billing insurance companies for their services. At times, clients will seek treatment massage in the wellness venues for many reasons—they are already a client or have friends who are clients—and you, as the therapist, will be called upon to SOAP chart. Once you begin communicating regularly with referring providers and insurance companies, the larger *Hands Heal* will be your best resource for ensuring steady reimbursement and a flow of referrals.

Pedagogical Features and Resources

Many stories, exercises, and quotations are included to enhance learning. In keeping with the native southwestern designs used in *Hands Heal*, I have assigned the following symbols to identify the three categories:

- Story Teller (Stories)—The story teller, weaving tales of the ancient ones, invites you to learn from those who came before.
- Bone Game (Exercises)—The dice, carved from the bones of animals, invite you to learn through play.
- Wise One Speaks (Quotations)—The wise, old owl invites you to learn through the wisdom of others.

Throughout the book, important words appear in bold type and important phrases are italicized. The boldface glossary terms are defined in the margins and are positioned directly across from the words as they are used in the chapter text. The italicized phrases represent what can be written on the Wellness and SOAP charts.

In addition to these features, the third edition text is accompanied by a Resource CD-ROM containing the following useful study aids:

- Quiz Bank—The Quiz Bank provides questions that readers can use to review material from each chapter and self-check their progress and comprehension.
- Quick Reference Abbreviation List—This convenient reference will assist readers with learning and using abbreviations common in documentation.
- Forms—The CD includes all of the blank forms that appear in the book. These can be printed and used for class activities or in professional practice.

Teaching Resources

An Instructor Resource CD-ROM is also available to instructors, and includes the following components:

- Instructor Manual—The Instructor Manual is organized into lessons that correspond with the chapters in the textbook. The lessons explore four categories of information: communication, documentation, insurance billing and ethics.
- PowerPoint Slides—The PowerPoint Slides provided on the CD are designed to assist instructors in presenting lecture material.
- Brownstone Test Generator—The Brownstone Test Generator contains a full bank of questions that instructors can use to create exams. The program allows instructors to add, delete, and otherwise customize the test questions to construct unique exams. The test bank includes questions that require the student to demonstrate knowledge and comprehension, as well as apply, analyze, synthesize, and evaluate information.
- Hands Heal Forms—The CD includes an array of blank forms that can be photocopied and distributed to students for use in class exercises.

The Instructor Resource Materials from the CD-Rom can also be accessed on *The Connection Web Site* at http://connection.lww.com/go/thompsonessnt.

Health care is evolving and people are increasingly proactive in their treatment choices of wellness care. The massage profession must stay up-to-date. You will find *Hands Heal Essentials* to be current, comprehensive, and critical to bridging health care and wellness care.

User's Guide

Hands Heal Essentials: Documentation for Massage Therapists is devoted to the "how and why" of charting wellness sessions. It is a complete learning resource that will help you understand the intricacies of documentation for massage therapy. This User's Guide shows you how to put the book's features to work for you.

CHAPTER OUTLINES

Each chapter opens with an outline that offers you a guide for material in the chapter.

BONE GAME BOXES

present activities and exercises that help you apply concepts and retain the material.

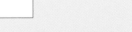

BONE GAME
Share Information During a Relaxing Foot Bath!

Initial interviews may extend beyond a half-hour for adequate information gathering. A foot bath is a creative way to keep your clients relaxed and the information flowing. If they think they are missing out on precious treatment time answering questions, they might tighten up the lips. A foot bath is one way to ensure that the client is comfortable and feels that therapy has already begun.

To provide a foot bath in the initial interview, prepare two plastic dish tubs—one with hot water; one with cold. Before inviting the client to select a tub, find out whether any health conditions would preclude benefit from either water temperature. If no contraindications are present, invite the client to choose one, or alternate between them, or scoop water from one tub to the other to obtain the preferred temperature. Tailor the foot bath by providing marbles to roll around underfoot or by adding essential oils. Have towels available within reach so the client can remove his or her feet from the bath at any time.

CHAPTER **3**

Documentation: Intake Forms

---

tegorizing like modalities: Massage Therapy—97124—is defined as massage, including . . . like effluerage, petrissage, and tapotement (such as stroking, compression, or percus- . . .). The purpose of the terminology is to provide a uniform language that will describe . . . lth care services accurately and will be an effective means for reliable, nationwide com- . . . nication among providers, patients, and third parties. However, there is no standard . . . rminology defining a style of massage: wellness, treatment, therapeutic, or medical. If . . . u choose to delineate different fees for these "styles" of massage, do so with a clear def- . . . nition and make sure that the specific modalities used do not overlap.

Another method for setting your fee schedule is to charge by time rather than by single code. This method is known as **bundling** services. Determine a set fee that includes any massage therapy applied. For example, you may use Swedish massage, myofascial release, lymph drainage, trigger point therapy, acupressure, and muscle energy techniques in varying combinations if you find it difficult to break them down into time per modality. You can choose to define your services using the general massage therapy procedural code—97124—and not bother with four different procedure codes and four different rates. Bundling services is common in cash practices and can be used with a billing practice as long as you are not bundling procedures that would be reimbursed at a lower rate than the one under which you are billing. This practice is known as **upcoding**.

bundling: type of reimbursement arrangement that combines two or more health care procedures into one procedure code

upcoding: process of increasing a CPT code from one of lower value to one of higher value that results in a higher reimbursement rate

Office Policies

Provide written statements of your office policies. Make sure your clients read them and agree to abide by them. Require a signature demonstrating that clients have read and understand your policies. It is easier to enforce something that is written down, signed, and dated. Keep the signed form in their file. You may have to remind your clients of these policies at a later date.

Cancellation policies are common in practices in which one session makes up a significant percentage of the daily income. Set a standard cancellation fee or charge the full price of the session if the client fails to cancel within a specified number of hours before the scheduled time. Consider abiding by your own cancellation policy. For example, offer a similar discount to those clients whose appointments you cancel without a 24-hour notice, or a "free pass" for a late cancellation in the future.

TERMINOLOGY

Key terms to know and understand are bolded in the text and fully defined in the margin.

STORY TELLER BOXES

share light-hearted anecdotes related to the content you just read.

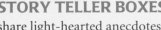

STORY TELLER
Listen With Your Hands

Aisha came in for her monthly session after the holidays and was bubbling with stories of her festivities. After chatting for a moment, I asked her, "What do I need to know to be of service to you today?" She replied that she was fine and couldn't think of anything to tell me. I struggled for a moment to release her respiratory diaphragm and asked her again. Again she replied that she couldn't think of anything. As she said that, her abdominal muscles tightened even more. I informed her that her belly was tighter than usual, but with her holiday glow, it sounded as though there was no stress in her family or social life. I asked her if anything unusual was going on at work. "The mayor is coming!" It was as though she was just remembering. She was in charge of a community service program and had spent the entire week preparing for the mayor's visit on Monday. Her stress level was over the top, and she put the site visit out of her mind to cope. Her body hadn't forgotten. She acknowledged that it was Friday, that there was nothing else to do, and that she felt prepared for the event. As she spoke about her week at work, her abdominal muscles softened and her diaphragm released. She admitted she could now relax, and she did.

WISE ONE SPEAKS
offer insightful quotes from professionals.

SAMPLE FORMS
Completed sample forms demonstrate
correct documentation procedures.

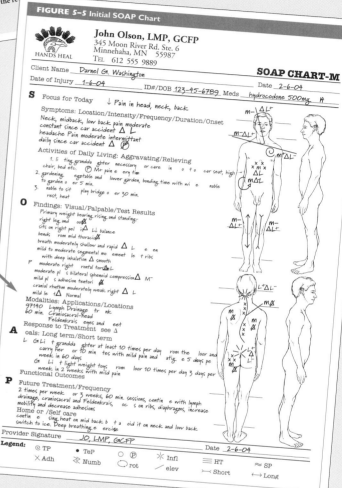

FIGURE 5–5 Initial SOAP Chart

CHAPTER SUMMARIES

reiterate the key concepts of the chapter and
offer suggestions and tips for practice.

SUMMARY

Developing the therapeutic relationship is central to the interview process and is even more important than gathering information or accurately assessing the client's condition. Trust, compassion, and understanding are the cornerstones of a productive relationship. Your ability to be fully present for your clients and to exhibit faith in their strength and healing abilities help lay these cornerstones in place. Without a strong bond, clients are reluctant to share their concerns, and treatment planning becomes a guessing game.

Concentrate on building the therapeutic relationship while striving to achieve the goals of the interview. Your tasks include:

1. Create a relationship.
2. Share information.
3. Develop goals for health.
4. Select and implement solutions.
5. Evaluate progress and provide feedback.

Communication is critical to achieving the goals of the interview. Employ the following verbal and nonverbal skills:

◆ Door-openers, open-ended questions
◆ Active listening: reflecting, paraphrasing, summarizing
◆ Complimenting
◆ Body language, including eye contact, posture, gestures
◆ Silence
◆ Touch

BONUS CD-ROM

The CD-ROM packaged with the book includes the blank forms from the book to use in practice, a Quick-Reference Abbreviation List, and a Quiz Bank for effective self-testing.

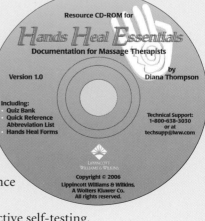

Acknowledgments

To all of you who generously shared your stories, appreciation, and feedback at conventions and workshops, thank you for providing much of the material for this edition of *Hands Heal Essentials*.

Thank you to Kerry Ann Plunkett, Eileen Stretch, ND, and Alternáre Health Services for the opportunity to embrace the needs of managed care documentation. Thanks also to Diane Hettrick and Bob May, ND, from Alternáre and Christine Carpenter from Regence.

A special thanks to Lori Bielinski and Deborah Senn (Washington State Insurance Commissioner) for your dedication to complementary medicine and for setting national precedence in complementary and alternative health care integration; and the law firm of Adler◆Giersch PS for its commitment and service to massage therapists. Without its work, there would be little need for this book.

I offer my warmest respect and heartfelt thanks to the people who made this book possible: my guardian angels Richard Adler and Lisanne Yuricich who taught me what I know and gave me the opportunity to share it; the staff at LWW who raised the ante on professionalism and quality; and my reviewers whose brilliant insights shaped the final product; Duane Hobbs, the designer of the new forms; Lori and Janelle Otterholt for assistance with the glossary; and Coleen Rene for the energy charting consult.

New to the *Essentials* edition is my editing team from Hearthside Publishing: Anne Seitz and Diane Geesey. Thanks for your leadership and playful spirits. You both possess a rare gift—the ability to support, manage, and put the person before the project. Thank you.

Reviewers

The publisher and author gratefully acknowledge the many professionals who shared their expertise and assisted in developing this textbook, appropriately targeting our marketing efforts, creating useful ancillary products, and setting the stage for subsequent editions. These individuals include:

Joanne Braun, BSEd, LMT
Educator
Owner, Tranquil Touch Therapeutic Massage
Kinnelon, New Jersey

Nancy W. Dail, BA, LMT, NCTMB
Director, Downeast School of Massage
Waldoboro, Maine

Josh Herman, ATC-L, LMBT
Miller-Motte Technical College
Massage Therapy Instructor
Cary, North Carolina

Stephanie Kacena, LMT
Nationally Certified—Massage and Bodywork
Director of Operations, Carlson College of Massage Therapy
Stone City, Iowa

Mary Reis, BA, LMT
Licensed Massage Therapist
Gainesville, Florida

Wendy L. Stone, MS, LMT
Chair, Pathology Department and
Practice Development Department
Muscular Therapy Institute
Cambridge, Massachusetts

Tomi Lynn Wilson, LMT
Portland, Oregon

Contents

CHAPTER **1**

Communication and the Therapeutic Relationship

CHAPTER OUTLINE

*T*he Creator gathered all of creation and said, "I want to hide something from the humans until they are ready for it. It is the realization that they create their own reality."

The eagle said, "Give it to me, I will take it to the moon."

The Creator said, "No. One day they will go there and find it."

The salmon said, "I will hide it on the bottom of the ocean."

"No. They will go there, too."

The buffalo said, "I will bury it on the plains."

The Creator said, "They will cut into the skin of the earth and find it even there."

Then Grandmother Mole, who lives in the breast of Mother Earth and has no physical eyes but sees with spiritual eyes, said, "Put it inside them."

And the Creator said, "It is done."

(A story from a Sioux friend told to Gary Zukav, author of *The Dancing Wu Li Masters and Seat of the Soul*. Reprinted with permission from Zukav G. In search of the soul. Life 1997;12:16.)

Let's change one word in this poignant story and pretend the Creator said, "It is the realization that they create their own *health*." The change does little to affect the message, yet this new twist proposes a powerful and significant concept for massage therapists and clients to consider: Individuals possess the ability to heal themselves. In reality, we exercise that ability every day—when we make simple decisions about what to eat, or seek care when we need it, or survive against overwhelming odds. All of us possess a life force that is tenacious and enduring, undiminished until the moment of our death. That life force drives us toward health.[1]

Therefore, clients may be the best people to involve in the healing process. Clients have all the data, take all the risks, and implement much of the solutions. When actively involved in their own healing, clients develop their self-confidence and sense of responsibility and become less dependent on their caregivers.[2] Our role as health care practitioners must expand to include providing our clients with opportunities for self-discovery, illuminating and expanding their unique strengths, tapping into their internal wisdom, and empowering them to heal themselves.

Introduction

In the past, the interview was used only to gather information about a client's symptoms and health history. The medical model demanded that the expert—the physician—collect data that would lead to an accurate assessment of the client's condition. Once a diagnosis was assigned, the standard of care for the client's disease was administered.[3]

Today, allopathic and alternative health experts recognize the flaws inherent in the traditional approach. First, human beings are individuals and respond uniquely to identical treatments. Second, a growing body of evidence indicates that emotions are responsible, at least in part, for disease. Some researchers believe that 90 to 95% of all clients who visit physicians have physical symptoms that are directly caused by emotions.[4]

Consequently, the central focus of the interview process has shifted from collecting data to building relationships. Health care providers from all disciplines embrace the client–practitioner relationship as their primary asset. One provider purports that the relationship *is* the therapy.[5] Some claim that trust is imperative for client satisfaction and compliance; others assert that trust or lack of it affects the results of any care provided.

Cardiologist Herbert Benson writes, "Belief or faith—whether it's deep in the mind or heart or focused on some outside object, like a physician—can play a key role in generating a response in the body."[4]

Trust is the key component to building meaningful relationships. Once the bond of trust is formed, clients will confide in us, provide us with insight into their conditions, and lead us to solutions that fit their lifestyles. Trust is established when clients feel understood. Until clients believe that the practitioner really understands what they are trying to say, clients are unlikely to believe that the practitioner has their best interests at heart or can be of any use to them. In the book *Kitchen Table Wisdom* by Rachel Naomi Remen, Dean Ornish, MD, puts it like this:

> Providing people with information—facts—is important but usually not sufficient to motivate them to make lasting changes in diet and lifestyle. If it were, no one would smoke. We need to work on a deeper level . . . to create a place safe enough for people to talk about what's really going on in their lives, to tell their stories, without fear of being judged, abandoned or criticized. Then, when people are really heard, are they likely to make lifestyle changes. (Reprinted with permission from Remen RN. Kitchen Table Wisdom: Stories That Heal. Riverhead Books: New York, 1996.)

This chapter first presents the communication skills massage therapists need for building relationships with their clients and includes exercises for developing those skills. It then describes the goals of interviewing clients and recommends approaches for reaching those goals. Entire books have been written on interpersonal communication skills and interviewing skills. This chapter introduces these two huge topics, but more importantly, it encourages readers to explore these complex subjects further. Good communication skills are essential to the therapeutic relationship and to good recordkeeping. Some of these skills may sound simple, but they are much more difficult to incorporate effectively than they appear. Practice by role playing with peers, performing the exercises in this book, attending workshops that will advance your communication skills, and reading books devoted to the subject. Invest as much time and energy in mastering communication as you devote to advancing your massage techniques. A suggested reading list is provided in Figure 1-1.

FIGURE 1-1   Resources for Communication Skills

1. *Kitchen Table Wisdom: Stories That Heal,* by Rachel Naomi Remen (Riverhead Books, New York, New York, 1996).

2. *Interviewing for Solutions,* by Peter DeJong and Insoo Kim Berg (Brooks/Cole, Pacific Grove, California, 1998).

3. *Messages: The Communications Skills Book, Second Edition,* by Patrick Fanning, Matthew McKay, and Martha Davis (New Harbinger Publications, Oakland, California, 1995).

4. *You and Me: The Skills of Communicating and Relating,* by Gerard Egan (Brooks/Cole, Monterey, California, 1977).

5. *The ABCs of Effective Feedback: A Guide for Caring Professionals,* by Irwin Rubin and Thomas Campbell (Jossey-Bass Publishers, San Francisco, California, 1997).

6. *People Skills: How to Assert Yourself, Listen to Others, and Resolve Conflict,* by Robert Bolton (Simon & Schuster, New York, New York, 1979).

7. *The Psychology of the Body,* by E. Greene and B. Goodrich-Dunn (Lippincott Williams & Wilkins, Baltimore, MD, 2004).

Interpersonal Communication Skills

A successful relationship with clients requires a variety of verbal and nonverbal communication skills. When you—the therapeutic professional—develop and use these skills, you lead clients to discover and accomplish their goals for health. You can enhance client cooperation and motivation, not by overcoming client resistance but by offering practical feedback that invites clients to focus on their strengths rather than on their pain. The interviewing skills introduced in this chapter will not only assist you in gathering information for treatment plans, but will also help your clients change their attitudes and summon the strength and wisdom to heal on a deeper level.

Here are detailed examples of various communication techniques that promote successful relationships with your clients.

BE PRESENT

No person can fully comprehend another, but with practice, guidance, and self-awareness anyone can learn to talk with a client. Talking may seem simple, but a great deal of skill is needed to be present with someone, especially a person in need. Pain often makes a person feel vulnerable and weak, and they may become anxious about taking risks and sharing personal information. It has been estimated that, without realizing it, people inject communication barriers—such as becoming argumentative, beating around the bush, or withdrawing—into their conversations more than 90% of the time when one or both parties has a problem to be dealt with or a need to be fulfilled.[2] A commitment to be present and available for your clients is the first step in manifesting trust and respect, which are the cornerstones of any productive relationship.

Being fully present for each client can be nearly impossible at times. We, as therapists, can get distracted—for example, by the last client who just suffered a tragedy, or the afternoon lecture we are rehearsing nervously in our mind, or the menu for tonight's dinner. We may habitually jump to conclusions and come up with a quick fix for a minor problem, while the deeper concerns are yet to be uncovered. Or we may make quick and easy value judgments based only on a client's appearance or hear a familiar situation in the client's words and filter the information through our own experience. Or we may show up with a personal agenda—the drive to succeed, a desire to contribute, an eagerness to practice new techniques or to try out new theories—and forget to honor our clients' role in their own health. We are all human. These distractions are normal. The important thing is to make a commitment to being present. Notice when you are distracted and bring your attention back to the person in front of you.

More should be done than feigning interest in our clients' stories. Whenever we offer anything less than our authentic self, clients can see right through. Robert Bolton, PhD, in his classic book *People Skills*, rates genuineness as the most important quality of communication and defines it as being open and honest, present and authentic. The keys to being genuine, as defined by Bolton, are self-awareness, self-acceptance, and self-expression. By cultivating these personal attributes, we will develop the skills necessary for being present and authentic with our clients.[2]

Here are some concrete tools and practical exercises for developing personal presence:

Self-Awareness

In today's fast-paced world, there is little time to sit still. We keep ourselves so busy that we often seek out experts to tell us who we are and what our purpose is in life. Self-help seminars and how-to books are numerous. We don't have time to explore our own ideas or to wait until the answers to our questions present themselves. The quick-fix attitude is everywhere.

On the other hand, self-awareness is not something found only on a mountain top or after years of meditation practice. It really can be found inside each of us—with a little practice. A simple way to develop our self-awareness is by listening to our inner voice.[2] If we are to trust in our clients' internal wisdom, we must learn to recognize our own. We must first acknowledge that we have a sense of inner direction, or intuition, and that we can trust it. Trust in our own intuition is strengthened with practice. We need to make time to listen to ourselves. We regularly tune out our internal voices or ignore them when they do surface by overworking, watching TV, or engaging in habits such as eating, drinking, exercise, and so on. Instead, we can get to know ourselves by spending a small amount of time each day being silent. With practice, we will begin to hear the voices inside us and distinguish where they are coming from. Some may be the voice of our mothers or of past experience, but the voice that softens the belly when it speaks is the voice of our intuition. Our "gut instinct" is literally just that. In Chinese medicine, it is believed that the stomach is the original brain.[10]

Practice using your intuition by placing your hand on your belly during your silent time and asking yourself yes or no questions. If your belly tightens, the answer is no; if it softens, the answer is yes.

▼

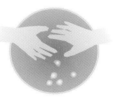

BONE GAME
Separate Self from Clients

Take five minutes between client sessions to breathe, stay silent, and be with yourself. It may be helpful to sit in a quiet, dark room with no distractions. During this time, mentally separate from your last client. You may need to run through the events of the last session and experience the feelings you may have chosen not to express in front of the client. A medical intuitive told me that in order to separate from the previous client, say silently or aloud, "I separate myself entirely—mentally, physically, spiritually, and emotionally—from Darnel. I call back all my energy, and I send him back all his energy."

When you have completed a session, check how you feel. Often, the lines blur between our clients' thoughts and feelings and our own. Be clear about who you are, separate from those you interact with throughout the day. Verify your feelings about the day, your work, and your health. Take a few deep breaths and feel the air move into your body. Notice how your body moves to accommodate the air as you breathe in and out. Imagine that the air moving through you is a life force, a warm light pushing life into every nook and cranny of your body. Experience your physical self and your emotional self.

Finally, prepare for the next client by inviting your internal wisdom to surface during the session. The Upledger Institute, in the CranioSacral Therapy seminars,

(Continued)

BONE GAME *(Continued)*

refers to internal wisdom or inner voices as your "inner physician." You may have other ways of referring to your intuition, in accordance with your belief system. If there is something you need help with, ask for specific guidance. Maybe you want the strength to refrain from judging Sara when she doesn't do her homework exercises or the confidence to listen to your intuition when you see Clint tense up when he reports he is fine. Affirm your self-awareness skills by saying, "I am whole and separate from Sara. I practice with skill and provide care that honors Sara as a whole and separate human being. It is my heartfelt intent to be present with Sara, to offer her my understanding and compassion, and to facilitate her healing by tapping into her strength and internal wisdom."

Self-Acceptance

Self-acceptance is about recognizing all aspects of our character, embracing our humanness, and trusting that we are enough. Self-acceptance is not synonymous with self-approval. It is not about ego. It does not mean we have to feel good about our behavior when we are hurtful. Self-acceptance begins by simply recognizing that all of us contain parts we may consider negative or even frightening. When we do not accept the full range of our feelings and thoughts, we often ignore our inner voice.[2] Fear and denial prevent us from understanding and relating to our intuition. It is impossible to separate the good from the bad, to love one and hate the other. Rachel Naomi Remen, MD, attended a seminar of Carl Rogers and reported him saying, "I realize there's something I do before I start a session. I let myself know that I am enough. Not perfect. Perfect wouldn't be enough. But that I am human, and that is enough."[6] When we begin to accept ourselves as being enough, we are able to be present for others.

An essential part of the individual healing process has to do with going within, into the shadow aspects—the aspects that, out of fear, we have denied, disowned, or suppressed. Shakti Gawain, in the book *Healers on Healing*, writes that the reason thoughts or feelings take a negative turn is because we do not accept them or allow them their natural expression.[6] Suppressed anger, for example, may manifest later as violence toward others or toward ourselves in the form of illness. If we can accept the good and the bad in ourselves, we will be better able to accept the positive and negative aspects of our clients. Start with yourself; kindness to others begins with kindness to yourself.

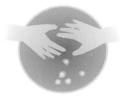

BONE GAME
Practice Acceptance

Exercise your ability to recognize a variety of human behaviors or characteristics in yourself.

Pick a day, preferably one with a full client load. You may have a few clients who push your buttons. If so, pick a day when they have appointments scheduled. If you are in school, use conversations with your classmates for this exercise. The task is to observe the conversations with your clients and notice when your "judgment flag"

(Continued)

BONE GAME *(Continued)*

waves, such as when the client does or says something about which you form a negative opinion. Throughout the day, take time to consider these observations. It is possible to do this exercise and still be present for your clients. Make a mental note of the
experience or jot down a reminder word on a sticky note.

Later that day, take a moment to review the situations that raised the judgment
flag. Pull out all the sticky notes and lay them out before you. Give yourself permission to be honest and compassionate with yourself. Hold up the proverbial mirror
and consider whether you have any of the traits you found fault with in your clients.
Remember, a mirror should reflect a clear image, not a sermon.

Repeat this exercise on another day, replacing the judgment flag with the times
when you felt admiration for the person before you. Again, make mental or physical
notes reminding yourself of the situations and review them later in the day. Consider
how you might find yourself in their stories.

Practice several times to strengthen your ability to accept all aspects of yourself.
You will then experience deeper compassion for others as well.

Self-Expression

Self-expressive people are aware of their innermost thoughts and feelings. They accept them,
and, when appropriate, they share their thoughts responsibly. In a client–practitioner relationship, it is rarely appropriate for the manual therapist to divulge his or her personal
thoughts or feelings. A rule of thumb is to share only the information that contributes to
the healing relationship. Self-expression is not self-disclosure. It takes a practitioner with
a developed sense of self-awareness and self-acceptance to know how to express the true
self without revealing personal information.

For example, talking about yourself can distract the client. Even though you may intend to create a true healing relationship, in which both heal and both are healed, clear
roles must be maintained. The therapeutic relationship requires the practitioner to focus
on the needs of the client. Be whole and complete with your clients without relating your
opinions or life events.

Self-expression can be relayed through a genuine interest in the client. One of the basic premises in Dale Carnegie's *How to Win Friends and Influence People* is that friends are
made when we become interested in others, not when we try to get others interested in us.
He even goes so far as to say, "It is the individual who is not interested in his fellow men
who has the greatest difficulties in life and provides the greatest injury to others."[7] Avoid
imposing on your clients by making them feel they have to take care of you. For example,
resist telling clients that your day got off to a rough start. That information may lead them
to filter their own needs and not make your bad day worse. Allow them their own process,
and keep yours to yourself.

You can demonstrate your interest in clients by listening to them—with your whole
body—and by watching their whole bodies and not just listening to their words. Many researchers claim that only a small portion of the understanding one gains from face-to-face
interactions comes from words. The results of these studies vary slightly. For example, the
importance of verbal information ranges from 7 to 35%, with the rest belonging to nonverbal communication.[2] Be conscious of your facial expressions. Surprise, alarm, worry,
distaste, or annoyance will steal across one's face and should be avoided. Give credence to
the expressions that steal across your client's face.

The therapeutic relationship is not an appropriate context for talking about yourself, but that does not mean you should suppress your thoughts and feelings completely. During the five minutes of quiet time between clients, feel those feelings, have those thoughts, and make those faces. Or designate a person with whom you can express your feelings at the end of the day or week. During the session, focus on the client's feelings. Be so clear in your own thoughts and feelings that you can reflect the client's words and expressions without distortion. One of the most productive interview skills is that of mirroring for clients, reflecting their innermost thoughts and feelings so that they may realize their inner wisdom. Avoid mirroring their negative thoughts. Instead, focus on reflecting their strengths. It is important to show understanding and compassion for their negative thoughts, but concentrate on reinforcing the positive ones.

Consider the potential obstacles to listening during the interview. Earlier, we discussed how easily practitioners can be distracted. Remember, it is very hard to listen when you are talking. Instead of talking about yourself, ask open-ended questions that elicit information about the client's situation. Find out how the client feels about the situation and how it is affecting his or her life.

▼

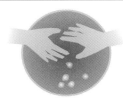

BONE GAME
Morning Pages

The best way I have found to get to know myself is to write three pages of whatever comes to mind, every morning, no excuses. This writing is called morning pages, a term I much prefer to "journaling," which feels so formidable and permanent. I learned of morning pages in Julia Cameron's *The Artist's Way*. I scribble thoughts, feelings, opinions—anger, grief, and desire—gossip, reactions to television shows, and movie critiques onto those pages, thus sparing my friends, loved ones, and clients. Writing morning pages has helped me sort out emotions and situations and has allowed me to express myself in ways I can be proud of. I have fewer regrets since practicing my daily writing routine. That alone is worth every minute of "I don't know what to write this morning . . . ." Try it. You will be amazed at what you discover about yourself.

Reprinted by permission from Cameron J. The Artist's Way: A Spiritual Path to Higher Creativity. New York: Tarcher/Putnam, 1992.

PRACTICE UNDERSTANDING AND COMPASSION
Develop Good Listening Skills

To foster good listening skills during the interview, limit the distractions in the room. For example, turn off the phone ringer. Don't wear clothes that call attention to yourself. Arrange the room so that nothing is between you and your clients—for example, avoid sitting behind a desk or crossing your arms or legs. Be on the same level as your clients—don't sit on the table. Face clients and make solid eye contact. Sit on the edge of your seat. Be relaxed, yet alert and involved. Respect their personal space—three feet is considered a safe distance in American culture. Gesture during their stories—nod your head, smile, and show concern. Touch—appropriately and with permission—to express your compassion.

Listen to the Words and Acknowledge the Feelings

Understanding clients involves grasping both the content and the process of client communication. The content refers to what clients say; the process refers to how they say it, which includes their tone, body language, and facial expressions. As mentioned earlier, most information is communicated nonverbally. When we focus on the symptoms alone, we miss the clients' personal reactions to their condition; in essence, we miss the uniqueness of each individual. Information is all around us. Feelings are the energizing force that helps us sort our stimuli and use them effectively to shape and implement relevant action steps.[2] Remember, when the clients do not feel understood about the facts and the emotions they express, they will not trust the practitioner, and the therapeutic relationship is at risk. To strengthen the relationship, we must explore the client's feelings as we gather the data.

Although you should be attentive to your clients' feelings, do not analyze those feelings or attempt to cross over into a psychotherapeutic relationship until you are trained and licensed to do so. The goal is to understand how clients feel about their condition, because their feelings can help or hinder the healing process. Research shows that, for example, excessive amounts of norepinephrine and epinephrine are secreted when a person is aggressive and anxious. The arteries thicken, and the excess hormones cause blood vessels to constrict. The gradual rise in blood pressure can cause hypertension, stroke, or heart failure.[6] Unless the client's feelings—verbally or nonverbally expressed—are considered, understood, and reflected by the practitioner, recovery from disease can be an uphill battle.

Clients do not always express their feelings freely. In Western cultures, people tend to be private with their feelings. Often, experiences have trained clients to hide their personal feelings initially. Until your clients feel safe enough to express themselves, look for alternative ways to gather emotional information.

Body language is the best way to tap into the client's feelings. Research shows that words are best at communicating facts, but body language is the primary means of emotional expression. The behavior of a person—facial expressions, postures, gestures, and other actions—is an uninterrupted stream of information and a constant source of clues to the feelings the person is experiencing.[2]

Reflecting and active listening are tools that can be used to acknowledge emotions you see in a client's behavior, whether or not they are expressed verbally. **Reflecting** means repeating, paraphrasing, or summarizing the feelings the client has expressed either verbally or nonverbally. **Active listening** involves paying attention to the speakers' tone, body language, and facial expressions and nonverbally demonstrating a sense of caring and respect. Use your intuition to read body language whenever clients do not name their emotion. Watch for facial expressions, postures, and gestures; listen to voice tone, pitch, and volume. If you are not sure what the expression means to the client, consider what it might mean to you and reflect your interpretation for confirmation.

Until you feel comfortable reflecting, adopt the formula, "You feel (name emotion) because (name event or condition)."[2] Practice this formula with your peers until it becomes natural. Use the formula to summarize the information the client (peer) shares with you. For example, "You feel sad because pain prevents you from lifting your baby,"

body language: behavior of a person, including facial expressions, postures, gestures, and other actions; a primary system for expressing emotions

reflecting: communication tool using parroting, paraphrasing, or summarizing the information and feelings the patient has expressed verbally or nonverbally

active listening: communication tool that demonstrates to the speaker that he or she is being understood and respected; nonverbal attendance to the speaker's tone, body language, facial expressions, and the like

or "You feel frustrated because you cannot concentrate on your homework with the headaches." Or even, "You feel happy because you were able to garden for an hour without back pain."

Sometimes, clients' body language reflects something different from their words. Check by saying, "You say you are happy that you were able to garden for an hour without pain, but you look as though you are sad that the back pain is still a problem and is preventing you from gardening for longer." Another example is, "Clint, I heard you tell me that you feel fine today, but I can't help noticing that you are wearing your shoulders like a pair of earrings. Is it possible that you are carrying some tension in your shoulders today?" A little humor, when used with discretion, can help to loosen up clients. Speak with compassion, not with prodding.

Exploring or reflecting feelings can be a useful tool for the following:

♦ Making the client feel understood
♦ Helping the client become more aware of her feelings
♦ Encouraging the client to speak more about her feelings

silence: communication tool that allows a patient to sort out thoughts, take a short breather from the work at hand, or search deeper for answers to the practitioner's questions

While a client is expressing her feelings, use **silence** to explore her emotions further. Silence can uncover deep feelings. Don't complete the client's sentences or fill pauses with more questions. If given time to think, clients will often sink a little more deeply into their thoughts and will express the feelings or problems that lie beneath the surface. Too often, therapists make the mistake of focusing on the first thing that comes up in the interview when the source of the problem is deeper. Your use of silence will add to clients' satisfaction with the therapeutic relationship and to their feeling of being deeply understood.

following skills: communication tools, usually open-ended questions, used to discover how a patient views a situation, including how he or she feels about something in life, how he or she views an event, and who or what the patient feels is important

In the interview, explore the client's entire relationship with her condition, including when and why she experiences it, how the condition affects her daily activities and emotions, and what she is doing to cope with it. **Following skills** are listening skills that can be used to discover how clients view their situation. **Door openers**—invitations to talk—can get things started. These can be as simple as, "You are here because of shoulder pain while working on the computer. Tell me how you feel about this." Open-ended questions can deepen the search. For example, "What do you notice when your shoulder starts to hurt and you have a deadline to meet?" Reinforce the tools that work for clients by **complimenting** them on being active in their health care. For example, "What a good idea, to stretch while sitting at your desk! It decreases the pain and helps you feel more energized." Lead them to explore additional ways of handling their stress and promoting physical healing. For example, "What could you do to remind yourself to stretch regularly even before the pain begins?"

door-openers: communication tool used as an invitation to talk; open-ended questions

complimenting: communication tool used to reinforce behavior, such as a positive reaction or evaluation by the practitioner in response to the patient or a question that indirectly implies something positive about the patient

See Through the Other's Eyes

Compassion is another key component to the relationship. We want the client to feel understood but not judged. Compassion denotes respect for the client's point of view. When developing relationships, look through the eyes of the other person—through his or her historical, cultural, and emotional filters. To do this, we must set aside our own belief systems, judgments, and expectations about the outcome of the relationship. Respect the client's personal values and personal space and allow the client to be her own person. You will still experience your biases and filters, but you will also demonstrate a commitment toward understanding and compassion and can return your focus to what is important to the person in front of you.

▼

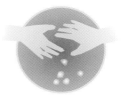

BONE GAME
Gain Perspective

Refer back to Bone Game: Practice Acceptance. After raising the proverbial mirror and considering the possibility that you may possess some of the same qualities as your client, add the following piece to the exercise:

Evaluate each situation separately. Put yourself in the shoes of each client. View the situation from the client's perspective, with his or her history and values, and see whether you can understand the motivations behind his or her actions.

To be compassionate is to be fair, patient, kind, and consistent. It is unconditional love—concern for the well-being of others—regardless of your opinion of them. From a Buddhist perspective, compassion is equal to emptiness. Pema Chödrön describes compassion as being soft and gentle, clear and sharp, open and warm.[8] A person with a well-developed sense of self-acceptance and has practiced kindness on herself will have an easier time feeling and expressing compassion toward her clients.

HAVE FAITH IN THE CLIENT'S STRENGTH AND HEALING ABILITIES

In the opening story of Chapter 2, a client named Sandee is having difficulty believing that her health is improving. Eventually, her massage therapist is able to illustrate Sandee's progress, convincing Sandee of the improvements. Providing substantial proof of her progress was like flipping a switch inside Sandee's head. Suddenly, she had confidence in herself and in the therapy and was willing to work harder to achieve greater results. Clients' perceptions, meanings, and definitions shift over time and in interactions with others. As practitioners, we must recognize that how we think, feel, and act greatly influences how our clients view their health.

According to research, people's perceptions of their own health can actually determine the quality of their health. People who feel hopeless about their situation or helpless to do anything about it generally have higher disease rates, are less able to fight infection and disease, and often will succumb to disease at a much higher rate.[4] Also, people who *feel* helpless have the same physiological response as people who *are* helpless: their heart rate slows, their blood pressure drops, the heart becomes prone to arrhythmia, the stomach pumps out less gastric secretion, and their urinary water and sodium decrease. The body secretes the stress hormone cortisol, which slows nervous system activity, decreases muscle tone, and suppresses immunity. The body behaves as though it is giving up.[4]

Encouraging clients to not give up—helping them believe that change is possible, even when they feel hopeless—is perhaps the most important thing massage therapists can do to help clients be successful in their efforts to heal. We must have faith in our clients, and in their ability to contribute to their own health.

The World Health Organization (WHO) defines health as "a state of complete well-being in all the aspects of one's life: physical, mental, social, and spiritual—not just the absence of disease."[4] The book *Mind/Body Health* provides a comprehensive list, shown here in Wise One Speaks: Qualities of Wellness. Use this list to develop ways to exhibit faith in your clients' strength and healing abilities and to influence the attitudes and emotions of your clients to promote improved health. If our attitudes influence our clients' perceptions of their health, thereby affecting the outcome, we should make it a point to influence their health in a positive way. When the mental, emotional, and spiritual aspects of wellness are manifested, the physical aspects follow naturally.

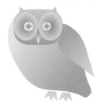

WISE ONE SPEAKS
Qualities of Wellness

- **Sense of empowerment and personal control:**
  –control over one's responses, not necessarily one's environment
  –integrity, the ability to live by one's deepest values
  –feeling heard and respected
- **Sense of connectedness and acceptance:**
  –to one's deepest self
  –to other people
  –to earth and the cosmos
  –to all regarded as good, and to the sources of one's spiritual strength
- **Sense of meaning and purpose:**
  –giving of self for a purpose of value; a caring sense of mission
  –finding meaning and wisdom in here-and-now difficulties
  –enjoying the process of growth
  –having a vision of one's potential
- **Hope:**
  –positive expectation
  –ability to envision what one wants before it happens

Reprinted with permission from Hafen BQ, Karren KJ, Frandsen KJ, Smith NL. Mind/Body Health: The Effects of Attitudes, Emotions, and Relationships. 2nd Ed. Boston: Allyn & Bacon, 1996.

Sense of Empowerment and Personal Control

Ensuring that clients feel heard and valued—an important component of the sense of empowerment and personal control—is a skill worked on previously in this chapter. In order for clients to feel heard, we as therapists must demonstrate that we understand what they say and how they feel. A variety of listening and communicating skills to help us do that have been introduced. We can express our understanding by creating a nondistracting environment in which we use body language to show we are listening, ask clients about their feelings, and reflect what we hear and see. By accepting what clients say without judging or criticizing, we show that we value what they are telling us.

We can help clients live according to their values by listening for what is really meaningful to them and integrating their values into the treatment plan. If Darnel is deeply committed to playing with his granddaughter and to showing her affection, but his low back pain prevents the types of activities he is used to, we can help him discover play activities that will not increase his discomfort (and possibly strengthen his low back in the process).

Once clients begin implementing self-care routines that are aligned with their core values, the contribution they are making to their overall goals for health is reinforced. Compliment them on their ability to affect their health, and they will feel they have some control over their situation. Provide options in your sessions regarding the types of massage available and educate clients on the various benefits of each option. This allows them to choose their treatment and self-care. A sense of control regarding the outcome of the massage sessions contributes to the speed and quality of recovery and allows clients to take responsibility and act effectively on their own behalf.

Lack of control may have an even stronger negative influence on health than having a high level of stress. Hypertension, anxiety, and pain levels increase, and the immune system is compromised. People who don't believe they can control or change their situation or who don't believe they are capable of contributing to their healing, slacken their efforts or give up altogether. Whereas, those who have a strong sense of control and ability exert great effort to master the challenge. Little effort on our behalf is required to compliment people on their contributions and to point out their successes.

Sense of Connectedness and Acceptance

Reflecting clients' words and feelings often helps them more clearly understand their situation, what it means to them, and how it fits into their life, even though all you may have done is summarize what they said. The information may seem new to them when they hear it put together for the very first time. This sense of understanding and being understood can help people feel a connection to the world.

Accept your clients for who they are and support their own self-acceptance. Your respect for their values gives them space to be who they are when they are with you.

Be an example for your clients. Demonstrate consistency by showing your respect for others. Be tolerant and flexible. Celebrate diversity. If you are critical of others in front of your clients, they may assume you are critical of them behind their backs. Have a positive attitude about yourself, your connection to others, your work, your profession, and the things that are meaningful to you.

Sense of Meaning and Purpose

No one is more valuable to the client than himself or herself, and nothing is more valuable than his or her health. One client made millions from the stock market through employee stock options and fully acknowledges that all the money in the world is not a substitute for health. Each client has only one body. Give your clients a sense of purpose by involving them in their healing process in a way that is satisfying and fulfilling.

Have your clients discuss the positives in their situation. When they believe something can be learned or accomplished from their pain, they are more able to muster up the courage to face it head-on.

Compliment your clients on their strength and wisdom and help them realize their unlimited potential to grow. Help your clients appreciate the process of growing and learning. They will have much to contribute to others after accomplishing the task at hand.

Hope

A positive expectation is the product of knowing what is possible and visualizing a positive outcome. When we help our clients understand how their condition is affecting them physiologically and how the body works to heal itself, they can visualize successful healing and support the results. Dr. Rachel Naomi Remen uses visualization to combat terminal diseases. In her book, *Kitchen Table Wisdom*, she tells the story of a client who used an image of catfish to enhance the function of his immune system and battle cancer. The client visualized " . . . millions of catfish that never slept, moving through his body, vigilant, untiring, dedicated, and discriminating, patiently examining every cell, passing by the ones that were healthy, eating the ones that were cancerous, motivated by a pet's unconditional love and devotion."[1] Dr. Remen compared bottom-feeders eating what does not support the life of an aquarium to white blood cells attacking and destroying cancer cells to help her client understand that his body was on his side. In the end, he was confident that the daily meditation contributed to his full recovery.

Hope is more than a positive expectation; it is the ability to fight against overwhelming odds and to laugh in the face of adversity. A fighting spirit has been shown to stimulate production of neuropeptides, which are chemical messengers that stimulate and mobilize the immune system. Humor dissipates stress and accentuates the positive. Laughter increases breath rate, circulation, and oxygen levels. Also, it relaxes muscle tension and breaks the pain-spasm-pain cycle—thus acting as a painkiller.

Physical health is only one aspect of wellness. Wellness includes mental acuity, a zest for living, and a tolerance for different ideas. Wellness brings with it empathy, compassion, and a sense of cohesiveness with the rest of humanity. Wellness encompasses a fighting spirit, an optimistic outlook, an attitude of hope. Take care of your clients' physical health, of course, but never omit the wholeness that is human. Whenever you can, maintain perspective, provide encouragement, boost clients' self-esteem, educate and provide options, prove that behavior can lead to positive outcomes, dispel doubts, encourage independence, and be flexible, consistent, positive, and responsive to your clients' needs. Do all this, and they will rise to the occasion and do much more for themselves.

Interviewing Skills: Team Therapy Model

Team Therapy Model:
paradigm for approaching the interview and information-gathering process; a combination of a medical model and intervention-free model of solution building

In this book, a new paradigm called the **Team Therapy Model** is proposed for approaching interviews. As holistic practitioners, we cannot entirely embrace the medical model, which implies that the expert's perceptions about the client's condition are more important than the client's perceptions. As massage therapists, we provide treatment and, therefore, cannot wholly adopt the intervention-free model of solution-building. Some massage therapists use touch as an additional form of communication, rather than for corrective purposes, as with the Rosen Method. Most massage therapy professionals, however, apply massage techniques with curative intent, whether for relaxation and stress reduction or to relieve pain and increase function. Therefore, a combination of the two models serves us best.

The primary goals of the Team Therapy Model approach to interviewing are:

1. Create a relationship
2. Share information

3. Develop goals for health
4. Choose and implement solutions
5. Evaluate progress and provide feedback

The rest of this chapter describes each goal and recommends methods for reaching it.

CREATE A RELATIONSHIP

Developing a deep and meaningful relationship that is productive for both client and practitioner is the primary goal of the interview process. This goal requires the practitioner to be mindful of the relationship from beginning to end. Creating and preserving a meaningful relationship calls for our constant attention, understanding, compassion, and faith in the client's personal strength and abilities. To foster such a relationship, practice the interpersonal communication skills described earlier in this chapter.

Countless opportunities exist for us to build productive relationships with our clients. The interview process is ongoing. It often begins before we meet the client (often through brochures and phone conversations) and extends beyond the time spent together. For example, the greeting on your answering machine can encourage or discourage the next step in initiating a relationship. For example, asking clients for permission to touch them and informing them of our intentions before massaging the chest may eliminate fear and open up potential for change, rather than resistance. Clients have described how, during times of pain or trauma, they heard their therapist's voice in their heads, instructing them to breathe, look, and listen for clues telling them how to take care of themselves. Relationships are developed before, during, and after every session, whether we are communicating actively or processing information indirectly. Make the most of these opportunities.

SHARE INFORMATION

Interviewing is an information-gathering process. Clients possess all the information you need, and you must simply create a trusting relationship in which information flows freely. Ask questions that lead to pertinent information and listen carefully to the replies. Every bit of information expressed by clients—verbal and nonverbal, symptoms and perceptions—leads to a deeper understanding of them and their health concerns, as well potential solutions. Grasping the relationship among the client, the condition, and the solution is the key to success.

According to Pema Chödrön, two primary obstacles to gathering information exist: thinking you already know the answer and being afraid to ask the question.[8] Proctoring countless practical examinations has shown me that it is human nature (or the product of watching television game shows) to leap to conclusions. We are so eager to solve the problem and to be the first to get the right answer that we don't take the time to thoroughly explore the possibilities or look beyond the obvious. We fall into what is most familiar to us. An examiner for a doctoral program in neurology explained that more than half the candidates failed the oral examinations, largely, he believed, because they didn't listen to everything the client said and therefore didn't obtain adequate information. They were too apt to focus on a key phrase or word that pointed to a familiar dysfunction. Instead, they should pursue lines of questioning suggested by the client's comments and gather additional information on which to base their conclusions.

▼

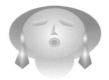

STORY TELLER
Explore Possibilities

I received a phone call from a chiropractor who was hosting a student apprenticeship program at her office. I was the faculty liaison. She called to complain that the student practitioner was treating all the clients as though they had rotator cuff injuries. Some clients did indeed have rotator cuff injuries, but others had thoracic outlet syndrome, carpal tunnel syndrome, or whiplash injuries. The student had recently studied rotator cuff injuries in a pathology and clinical treatment class. As a result, she was listening for familiar information and didn't bother to register other important information. Instead of exploring all possibilities, she jumped to the explanation that she had the most immediate information about: If the client had shoulder pain, it must be caused by a rotator cuff injury.

Solving minor problems while ignoring deeper concerns is one of the biggest sources of inefficiency in industry, government, schools, and health care.[2] We leap to conclusions because we are eager to help, want to be right, are in a hurry, or have any number of other reasons or motivations. We are desperate to explain our experience, so we force-fit a few pieces of information into familiar scenarios and call it good, rather than searching for more details without the pressure of categorizing the data. Sometimes, the process of asking questions and gathering information can be far more important than identifying a cause or pinpointing a dysfunction because it can lead clients to a better understanding of themselves, their relationship with their bodies, and their role in their own health.

Be more curious than afraid. Often, we avoid asking questions when we cannot control or anticipate the response. We are afraid of information we might not understand or feelings that could get out of hand. Someone's story might be more than we can handle, or we won't know what to do with the information once we know it. We fear the client will think we are asking silly questions or being nosy. If the question arises in your mind, and a part of you believes the answer could contribute to the client's health, trust your instinct and ask.

Other times, we avoid asking meaningful questions because we assume the client's intentions are simple. If we work in an environment where relaxation massage is paramount, for example, we may assume that the only reason for the client's visit is to relax or be pampered. We don't want to probe too deeply into their day celebrating Sue's birthday, so we avoid asking direct questions and automatically provide a routine session. A pointed question, such as, "Is there anything I should know about you that would help us reach your goals for health today?" could heighten their experience of your massage by inviting a deeper level of participation, which may ultimately lead to a session that satisfies specific health needs.

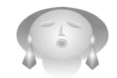

STORY TELLER
Be Curious

Do not let fear limit your ability to serve. I remember the first time a client cried during a session. I handed her a tissue and considered stopping the work I was doing on her legs because it seemed too emotionally difficult for her. I was afraid to break the silence and ask her about it. Eventually, I summoned the courage to say, "I see that you are crying. Shall I stop what I am doing, or would you like me to continue?" She said, "Oh no, please continue. I am crying because I have never been touched in such a respectful and caring manner before." I almost missed out on the most moving comment anyone has ever made about my work.

Explore the data thoroughly and include the client's thoughts, feelings, behaviors, and experiences. Reflect the content and the context of the client's story. Affirm the client's perceptions and your interpretations. Exploring and reflecting client perceptions is the most important aspect of interviewing skills. When explored and understood, these perceptions help therapist and client alike make sense of health issues and can lead to a better understanding of the relationship among the client, the client's condition, and the successful treatment.

What questions are important to ask? It is difficult to determine whether information is helpful before you know what the information is and get a sense of how the client feels about the information. Leading questions will follow a pre-determined path—yours. Open-ended questions allow for individual expression and interpretation from the client's point of view. Engage in conversation instead of asking an endless stream of questions. The conversation can begin with something as simple as, "Tell me about your health concerns," or "What are your goals for today's session?" Choose the significant details from the client's story and listen for clues that provide a direction for additional open-ended questions.

Prevent people from rambling. Create purposeful dialogue by interrupting with brief reflections of helpful information. A long-winded story may have one vital piece of information that can be paraphrased back to the client to break his chatter and to focus attention on providing deeper insight into the relevant detail.

Some clients have difficulty talking about their concerns or asking for what they want. Take your cues from the intake forms. Clients may find discussing their problems uncomfortable but have no trouble putting the information on paper. The difficulty may lie in your choice of language or your focus on a particular condition. To let the client lead you, ask, "What should I know today so we can meet your goals for health?" Compliment clients on what they have done for their own health—even showing up for the appointment. Compliments may help them open up.

Acquiring information from clients is an art. You will need to cultivate a flexible style to accommodate clients' differences in background, in knowledge about massage therapy, and in other health matters. It is important to use language that your client understands and to use consistent terminology. As you ask your questions, define the specialized terms you use. Avoid either speaking down to clients or speaking over their heads.

The Preinterview

Clients initiate the relationship by gathering information about you and determining whether you are the right massage therapist for them. Make sure your external image—ads, brochures, office space, and the like—attracts the type of client you are seeking. Identify your target clientele and speak directly to them in your marketing efforts and in the way you project yourself.

Once the client takes the next step and contacts you directly, gather enough information before scheduling the appointment to determine whether you want to pursue the relationship. Find out why the client is seeking care and get a few details about his or her health history, so you can decide whether you can and want to be of service or whether a referral is in order. Ascertain in advance whether you will need a doctor's prescription or consultation before treating the client so that the first session will not be a waste of time for either one of you.

In advance of the first appointment, share any information you feel is important for preparing clients emotionally and physically for the session. Explain what they can expect during the session, what the fees are, and what to wear, for example. Invite prospective clients to ask questions about your experience, modalities, education, affiliations, and references to assure them that they have made the right decision and to put them at ease. Be prepared to mail information to them prior to the first session, such as your credentials, office policies, intake forms, directions, and so on. Avoid confusion and limit the potential for unmet expectations.

The Interview

Gather information that helps the client relax, enhances the relationship, and opens the dialogue. Begin by asking how the client prefers to be addressed—Ms. Freeman? Karen?—and tell her how you prefer to be called. Chat a little bit to make her comfortable and to get to know her a little bit. For example, you might begin with: "It's a beautiful day today. Do you have plans to enjoy the weather?" Limit the sharing of personal information about yourself. For example, let them know you are looking forward to working in the garden, but don't delve into your plans for landscaping. Instead, place the focus on getting to know the client.

Review how you work and what the client can expect during the session. For example: "To begin with, I need to understand as much about your goals for health and your expectations of me as possible. In addition, it is helpful to explore how your past may be influencing today's concerns, so I may be asking you a lot of questions. All this can take a while, but I promise that you will get at least 45 minutes of hands-on therapy today. In the future, a couple of minutes may be all that's needed to get me up to speed before we begin the session." Even if you explained things over the phone, information can be received differently when people are face-to-face. Watch clients' reactions to your information and be responsive to their needs.

Initial interviews can be extensive and time-consuming, depending on the clients' health concerns. It is advisable to schedule time for the interview in addition to the treatment session or shorten the hands-on part of the session to allow for the extensive interview and to stay within the standard treatment time. The information obtained in the interview is critical to conducting safe and effective treatment, and it increases efficiency in the long run. Whether or not the client has vital medical information to share, it will be best to do a complete interview in the first session or two, rather than having information trickle in over time.

add Interview time + @ time (handwritten margin note)

Clients may have health conditions that make it difficult to sit for extended periods of time. Others may get antsy. Be attentive and responsive to their spoken and unspoken needs. Intersperse movement assessment tests with the question-and-answer format. Clients may want to begin the hands-on part of the session immediately. Be flexible and gather information with your client in sitting, standing, or lying positions. Make sure you have obtained adequate information before you begin treatment. Try juggling verbal questions with hands–on information gathering or relaxation techniques to keep the client comfortable. Avoid beginning therapy before you have enough information to provide safe treatment.

▼

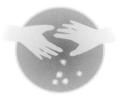

BONE GAME
Share Information During a Relaxing Foot Bath!

Initial interviews may extend beyond a half-hour for adequate information gathering. A foot bath is a creative way to keep your clients relaxed and the information flowing. If they think they are missing out on precious treatment time answering questions, they might tighten up the lips. A foot bath is one way to ensure that the client is comfortable and feels that therapy has already begun.

To provide a foot bath in the initial interview, prepare two plastic dish tubs—one with hot water; one with cold. Before inviting the client to select a tub, find out whether any health conditions would preclude benefit from either water temperature. If no contraindications are present, invite the client to choose one, or alternate between them, or scoop water from one tub to the other to obtain the preferred temperature. Tailor the foot bath by providing marbles to roll around underfoot or by adding essential oils. Have towels available within reach so the client can remove his or her feet from the bath at any time.

Review the intake form, find out what the client's goals and expectations are for the visit, and reflect the client's general goals for health and priorities for treatment. Ask, "How can I help you?" or "Why are you here?" Hearing the client speak adds to the written information on the form. It also apprises you of any inaccurate presumptions or unreasonable expectations and gives you an opportunity to change these instead of disappointing the client. Setting reasonable goals is essential to a productive relationship—a subject that will be discussed at length in this book. Begin the discussion by listening and comprehending the client's goals for health and for sessions with you. Later, move to shaping and developing the client's goals with the purpose of tracking outcomes and promoting client participation.

Explore the treatments the client has tried and the modalities he is considering. Ask "What worked or didn't work?" or "Do you have a sense of why the previous treatments did not work?" These questions will make your sessions more efficient because you can use treatments the client likes and believes are effective, rather than spinning your wheels with treatments that have already been proven ineffective.

Use the intake forms to begin a direct line of questioning regarding history and current conditions. Take note of your client's priorities and focus on them. You may be interested in her respiratory history, while she is intent on getting attention for a recent knee injury. Make the client feel that his or her needs are being met before focusing on less urgent details.

▼

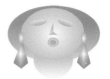

STORY TELLER
Memories Affect Healing

Explore relationships between current symptoms and previous history. Stimulate the client's memory to connect previous events such as traumas, illnesses, repetitive movements, and the like that may have initiated the current condition. Little things may trigger important memories. For example, as one client was watching a large family board an airplane, she noticed and identified with the eldest child's difficulty carrying a younger sibling. There were too many kids for the parents to take care of, so the older kids were helping with some of the younger ones. My client, too, was the eldest in a large family. Her mother had died when she was young, and she shouldered a great deal of responsibility in caring for her younger siblings. That memory, combined with the interview question, "What kinds of things did you do as a child that might have been stressful to your neck?" pulled it all together for her. She not only had a great deal of physical stress with her younger brothers and sisters clasping their hands around her neck to help her lift them, but she also carried the weight of the responsibility of trying to replace her mother. By recognizing the origin of the physical stress and acknowledging an emotional component, she reduced the occurrence of her neck spasms dramatically.

Explore the details of clients' health concerns. Prompt clients with consistent adjectives, such as mild, moderate, and severe, as you gather information. Using consistent terminology to describe, for example, the intensity of pain, will show progress more clearly over time. Comparing moderate pain with mild pain is easier than distinguishing between "hurts pretty bad" and "is kinda sore." The ability to demonstrate progress is an important component of documenting information—measurable data leads to measurable results. Let them know the importance of using consistent terminology and paraphrase the details they provide until they feel comfortable using the terms themselves. Soon, they will be saying, "I had a constant, moderate headache that lasted for two days and interfered with my ability to concentrate at work."

Information regarding the client's medications can be enlightening and helpful in creating a safe treatment plan. The list of medications on the intake form can be daunting at times. Keep a **Physician's Desk Reference (PDR)** handy to look up medications and their side effects. Better yet, ask the client for information. Find out why he is taking the medication. You may uncover a condition not listed on the intake form. Ask about side effects. Manual therapy has the physiological effect of increasing circulation and may increase the metabolic breakdown of the medication.[9] Be alert to an onset or increase in those side effects. (For general principles regarding safe massage choices for clients on medications, refer to Persad RS. Massage Therapy and Medications: General Treatment Principles. Toronto, Ontario: Curies-Overzet, 2001.)

Physician Desk Reference (PDR): resource manual of drugs and medications, in addition to information on generic terms, doses, and side effects

Hands-On Interview

The interview—asking questions, listening, and observing—segues into the hands-on interview—questioning the whole body, listening, observing, palpating, and testing. Make it a point to acknowledge that you are moving from hands–off information gathering to hands–on information gathering. The initial touch affects how the client will respond to subsequent physical contact. He or she may relax into your touch or pull away or be open to treatment or resistant to it. Ask clients for permission to touch them prior to your first hands-on contact. This demonstrates respect and instills trust. It can make the difference between feeling poked and prodded and being handled with compassion and caring. Tell clients where you are about to touch them and why you will be touching them there and ask for their consent before you follow through with the contact. You may need to do this for only a session or two. Once trust is solidified, you can obtain their permission to discontinue the consent questions.

Educate your clients throughout the hands-on interview. Prepare them to stand up, sit down, and walk this way before you put them through the paces. Let them know why you are palpating their neck, especially if it is their back that hurts. Tell them your goals for each modality and invite them to visualize the results you intend. Inform them of your options and allow them to choose the techniques you will use.

The interview and the hands-on interview involve verbal and nonverbal communication, and they may present you with conflicting information. You may hear the client say one thing, yet you may witness the opposite response in facial expressions or tension patterns. Reflect both findings when this happens and invite the client to make sense of the possible conflict. The client may be unaware of the contradiction. Presenting your findings in a neutral or curious way invites the client to work with you to resolve it. This promotes partnership and gives the client a deeper understanding of herself rather than putting her on the defensive.

▼

STORY TELLER
Listen With Your Hands

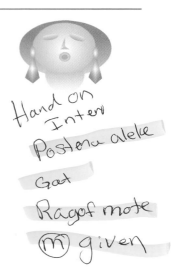

Aisha came in for her monthly session after the holidays and was bubbling with stories of her festivities. After chatting for a moment, I asked her, "What do I need to know to be of service to you today?" She replied that she was fine and couldn't think of anything to tell me. I struggled for a moment to release her respiratory diaphragm and asked her again. Again she replied that she couldn't think of anything. As she said that, her abdominal muscles tightened even more. I informed her that her belly was tighter than usual, but with her holiday glow, it sounded as though there was no stress in her family or social life. I asked her if anything unusual was going on at work. "The mayor is coming!" It was as though she was just remembering. She was in charge of a community service program and had spent the entire week preparing for the mayor's visit on Monday. Her stress level was over the top, and she put the site visit out of her mind to cope. Her body hadn't forgotten. She acknowledged that it was Friday, that there was nothing else to do, and that she felt prepared for the event. As she spoke about her week at work, her abdominal muscles softened and her diaphragm released. She admitted she could now relax, and she did.

Hands–on information gathering can take many forms, depending on the modalities used. You will use various techniques—palpation-assessing system integrity, postural analysis, motion testing, and the like—according to your individual specialty or training as a massage therapist. As you ask questions, the body responds as well as the voice. For example, in Upledger's CranioSacral training, practitioners are taught to listen for the truth in the body by asking questions and feeling for changes in the craniosacral rhythm as the client verbalizes answers. If the movement of the cerebral spinal fluid stops, the answer to the question is significant to the healing process. Develop your individual skills and gather adequate information for determining safe and effective treatment.

The hands-on interview is a mixture of information gathering, treatment, and evaluation. As new information presents itself, treatment shifts to comply. The effectiveness of the treatment application is immediately assessed, providing new data. The interview cycles continuously throughout the hands-on session. Be aware of this and don't reserve the information gathering for before and after only. If necessary, stop periodically throughout the hands-on session to record the information obtained. A Feldenkrais practitioner incorporates breaks into her sessions. Her invitation to rest for a few minutes gives her a chance to take notes without the client feeling that he or she is being ignored.

As you share the information you are gathering with your client, try not to reflect only negative findings. Saying "This is really tight" or "That feels very congested" over and over again can be discouraging. Instead of judging the client's joint mobility, ask him to describe what he feels. For example, "How does your shoulder feel when I move it like this?" Asking the same question after you have applied treatment can help integrate the solution, making a mental connection to the physical change. "Now how does your shoulder feel when I move it?" Compliment the client on his progress. Reinforce the work he contributes between sessions. "Your tissue feels great here. You must be very successful with your stretching routine."

Post-Interview

In the final stage of the interview process, summarize the information gathered throughout the session and confirm your findings with the client. Ask the client which treatment modalities and application locations felt productive and which ones were not so effective. Present your assessment of the client's progress and response to the treatment. Compliment the client on his or her participation during the session and verbalize your thanks for contributing to the outcome. By summarizing the information and drawing conclusions about the effectiveness of the treatment, you increase your client's awareness of the value of the session, make her conscious of the benefits, and acknowledge her ability to contribute to the outcome.

DEVELOP GOALS FOR HEALTH

So far, the focus has been on building productive relationships with clients and uncovering information that aids in providing safe and effective massage therapy. To be truly effective in producing ongoing results, however, we must understand our clients' needs and identify goals that direct the treatment plan and illustrate progress over time. The goals should be specific, measurable outcomes that the client and the practitioner strive to attain.

Health goals are hinted at early in the therapeutic relationship. During the initial consultation, clients describe the physical complaints and the desired results. Intake forms record their health concerns and goals for health. Throughout the interviews, the practitioner listens to the clients' needs, explores their symptoms, researches their history, and tries to understand the impact of the condition on their lives. This information empowers the practitioner to formulate goals to ensure that the clients' needs are met.

Pngese from fisec
1. carifi pigonss
2. Jcd9 code
   Riten order
3. tintmat desicties
   frcance dreats
   Haw ofte   long
4. do not cange
   state on city
      tay

When developing goals with clients, explore the following questions: How do your clients define wellness? What are their expectations of you and of themselves? How can you contribute to their vision of their own health?

Define Client Needs

First, focus on the needs of the client. Often, we have agendas based on what we think is best. We may see things that need fixing and be eager to impress our clients with our ability to treat their conditions. We may pressure people into fixing problems they are not emotionally or physically prepared to address. Behavioral scientists have noted that the less a person is under pressure from others to change, the more likely change will occur.[2] Therefore, we should fully understand our clients' needs and support them to accomplish their goals for health—when and how they choose. We do not have the final say on what is best for our clients.

We must help our clients articulate their needs. They may have well-formulated complaints but limited experience in transforming symptoms into goals. When needs become palpable, clients can identify significant, tangible goals. For example, Darnel complains of low back pain. He hopes the massage therapist will get rid of his pain. The goal—to eliminate the pain—can be intimidating and its pursuit frustrating for both the practitioner and the client. It is difficult to measure changes in pain, and it is nearly impossible for the client to experience progress—a decrease in pain—when the pain continues to be endured daily. Do not focus on pain when exploring the needs of the client. Instead, focus on function—how pain limits the client's ability to participate in daily activities. We are better able to comprehend the needs of our clients when we understand how their symptoms affect their quality of life.

Construct Functional Goals Based in Activities of Daily Living

Once we discover how our clients' symptoms are affecting their daily routines, we can formulate **functional goals** (or measurable goals) for health. For example, Darnel cannot pick up his granddaughter Madi and give her hugs because of the pain in his low back. Both Darnel and Madi are negatively affected by the loss of intimacy. Rather than selecting a goal based on a symptom—to eliminate low back pain, which is difficult to measure and problematic to experience accurately—develop a goal based on a function—such as lifting Madi and hugging her, which is of great importance to Darnel and his granddaughter. Take a significant activity the client is yearning to get back to and develop it into a well-defined goal that both you and he can strive to accomplish.

functional goals: short-term and long-term goals for health based on daily activities that the client is having difficulty performing

Functional goals are set by the client, with assistance from the massage therapist, to address the specific needs of his or her everyday life with the purpose of leading to an effective treatment plan. Goals must be specific to an activity of daily living and be measurable and achievable in a reasonable amount of time. The client and therapist can further define the functional goal by specifying the parameters for success. How often does the client want to perform the activity? What is a reasonable time frame for success? Will Darnel be satisfied when he can lift Madi five times a day but has to increase his pain medication as a result? A well-defined goal should reflect:

◆ Quantity, duration, or both—How much or for how long (duration)? What number of pounds to lift or stairs to climb three times a day or four hours a night (quantity)?
◆ Frequency—How often? Eight hours a day or five days a week?
◆ Quality—How are symptoms affected? Does the client awake feeling moderately fatigued or does he experience mild pain?
◆ Time frame—When will goal be accomplished? Is it within two weeks or by the end of the month?

A functional, measurable goal for Darnel might be to lift and hug Madi three times a day for five days a week and feel no more than moderate pain in his low back in a time frame of within 30 days.

Part of defining and developing goals with clients is to help them participate in life, look for alternative ways of living a quality life, and regain their ability to do the things they want to do. This is easily accomplished by setting short-term goals that they can achieve and by motivating them to stretch a little farther each week to get closer and closer to their goals for health.

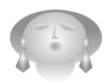

complementary and alternative medicine (CAM): medical and clinical services provided by practitioners that are not normally taught by conventional medical institutions; also includes providers whose services are not usually paid by traditional insurance programs

STORY TELLER
Functional Outcomes Prove Massage Efficacy

I gave a presentation at a symposium to 100 doctors on the integration of **complementary and alternative medicine (CAM)** and how to refer to massage therapy. A well-known researcher, Dr. Dan Cherkin, was scheduled to present his findings on the effectiveness of CAM care on chronic low back pain immediately after my talk. By way of introducing me, the moderator waived Dr. Cherkin's newly published research paper in the air, contending, "Can you believe these results? I'm sure you are as shocked as I am. Really, have you ever seen a SOAP chart from a massage therapist show that massage relieves pain anywhere?" Looking out over a crowd of physicians shaking their heads "no" was a humbling experience to say the least, but a telling one.

Unfortunately, the moderator was accurate in proclaiming that massage therapists' charts often do not adequately reflect the positive outcomes that result from our patient/practitioner relationships. I have reviewed thousands of SOAP charts from manual therapists as part of my work with insurance credentialing. It is rare that the charts reflect a cessation of pain. As a result, one could surmise that the treatment was ineffective. If, instead of focusing on the patient's pain, our charts recorded the patient's increased ability to perform daily activities, the 100 physicians at the symposium would have embraced the research results as affirming common knowledge.

functional outcomes: goals for which a client's progress toward improved health creates an increased ability to participate in daily activities

The key to our credibility lies in charting **functional outcomes**. Drs. Cherkin and Eisenberg demonstrated this very issue in research results: Massage therapy resulted in a statistically and clinically significant improvement in the ability of patients to perform their daily activities when compared with self-care exercises (P<.001). Massage was also more effective than self-care exercises in decreasing pain (P=.01), but the benefits were less pronounced.[10] These results are easily understood when you consider one's threshold of pain. People feel compelled to follow their routines—bathe, dress, work, exercise, garden, and play—and tend to stop only when they reach a certain level of pain. If we rely solely on charting pain, we are likely to see a steady level of pain over time, even when the patient reports improvement. Whereas charts that record a patient's ability to perform daily activities may reflect considerable progress toward his or her goals for health. Translate patient complaints into functional limitations and set measurable goals based in activities of daily living, and you will be able to clearly demonstrate progress as a result of your manual therapy sessions.

CHOOSE AND IMPLEMENT SOLUTIONS

Solutions encompass all of the following:

◆ The client's self-care routine and homework exercises
◆ The treatment provided by the massage therapist and other health care providers on the team
◆ Any belief, act, or intention that brings the client closer to the health goals already set

The term "solutions" is used to encourage client–centered treatment planning. Clients, their family members and friends, the spiritual figures they consult, and the health care team contribute to the client's expression of health. The important point in choosing and implementing solutions is to consult the clients and encourage their participation in all aspects of treatment.

Discover the client's strengths. Find out what she is already doing to take care of herself. Use questions about comfort, not pain, to discover the client's abilities to heal. Focus on the positive whenever possible. Too often we dwell on pain. We ask clients to chart their pain on intake forms; we question clients about their pain during the interview; we ask, "Does this hurt?" when we touch them. Instead of asking how frequently they experienced pain today, ask about when they felt good. Use this discussion to explore their strengths. Find out what was going on around them when they felt good. Did they do something that triggered that good feeling? Help them see how they contributed to the good feeling. Compliment them on knowing what to do to feel better, reinforce that activity as a solution to their condition, and encourage its use. If we are to involve our clients in their healing process, we must tap into the resources already available to them.

WISE ONE SPEAKS
Focus on the Positive

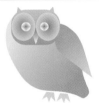

Consider this quote:

"When I focus on what's good today, I have a good day, and when I focus on what is bad today, I have a bad day. If I focus on the problem, the problem increases; if I focus on the answer, the answer increases."

Quotation attributed to Bill W. Alcoholics Anonymous.

Explore additional ways in which clients contribute to their own healing. Brainstorm solutions without clarifying, judging, or dismissing them. Be creative in the search and be open to different ideas. Share in the brainstorming by building on ideas the client has presented. The goal is to create homework and self-care activities that the client can successfully apply to improve his health. These discussions may take time in the beginning, but they will save time over the long run and can easily take place during the hands-on massage time. The discussions promote self-awareness and reinforce the concept that the client is capable of effecting his own well-being. The client will learn from this experience and explore other solutions between sessions. He or she will be forthright in offering ideas throughout the therapeutic relationship, thus saving the therapist from the process of trial and error. Failed attempts at homework assignments will be reduced because the homework will be the client's idea. Treatment applications will be welcomed because they were discussed and agreed upon in advance. Show respect for your clients and consider their input in all decision making.

Educate your clients on the effectiveness of various solutions. They may have several ideas that they are willing to implement but lack particular knowledge about when to use one option over another and how each option works. If clients understand when to try a particular exercise and how that exercise helps them attain their goals, they may be motivated to try it more often. Solutions fall by the wayside when their value is not realized. Teach clients how the body's healing mechanism works and demonstrate how their solutions affect their health. Invite them to imagine their body healing as they do their homework.

Narrow the list of possible solutions and discuss the pros and cons of those remaining. A long list of solutions can overwhelm the client. Select one or two to implement between now and the next session. Plan what, how, when, and where to do it. Remind the client how it works. Demonstrate proper applications of solutions and correlate them with other activities. For example, teach Darnel proper lifting techniques to prevent re-injury and promote recovery. Invite him to practice his new-found lifting techniques with his granddaughter and apply the same techniques to lifting groceries and laundry.

Be vigilant in pursuing client-centered solutions. Practitioner-imposed solutions are often unsuccessful. Too often, we classify clients as resistant or uncooperative when they do not follow through on assigned homework or self-care activities. Noncompliance is generally attributed to the client's personal flaws or to some deep-seated pathology. In the medical model, the professional is rarely, if ever, held responsible for the mismanagement of the therapeutic relationship. If the client shows progress, the practitioner can take the credit and feel competent, but the notion of client resistance lays most of the blame for lack of progress on the client and distances the practitioner from responsibility.[3] Steve de Shazer has proposed that what practitioners take to be signs of resistance are, instead, the unique ways in which clients chose to cooperate.[11] Keep in mind that it is your clients' choice to participate in their healing. Do not judge them if they are not successful in their efforts. Take responsibility. It is possible that you selected homework that doesn't fit their lifestyle instead of focusing on their unique healing abilities.

Don't give homework to clients who are not committed to change. Giving them tasks to do would only show that you are not listening to them. Instead, ask them to pay attention to occurences in their lives that tell them the condition can improve. Ask them to pay attention to the days that are better and notice what is different. Wait until clients are able to trust that their health can improve.

Encourage self-awareness before exploring solutions. Provide information and self-care education that heightens clients' awareness of their relationship with the condition. Help them listen and respond to the messages their bodies give them throughout the time between sessions. When clients are ready, teach them to pay attention to internal warning signs, such as tension in the shoulders, and to respond before their symptoms get out of hand.

Treatment Options

Treatment is a collaboration. When only one person in the therapeutic relationship is seen as the healer, fixing the problem may be possible, but healing is not. Although the client may benefit in some ways, he or she will be stuck in a dependent relationship, with little opportunity to experience strength and growth. Each of us has a technique—perhaps several—that we use to treat our clients. It is important to remember that the technique does not heal; the relationship does. The treatment you provide simply facilitates the client's own self-healing capabilities. Use the technique as another opportunity to listen to the client, to understand her, and to help her find her way toward better health.

Typically, clients defer to the expert practitioner regarding options for massage. They do not know the full scope of what is available, they do not have experience in the variety of techniques, and they do not understand the pros and cons of the options before them. None of these facts justifies leaving clients out of the decision-making process. Whatever your massage techniques, educate your clients on their advantages and disadvantages. During the interview, discuss the various places on their bodies that the techniques can be applied. Ask whether they have any preferences to the style of massage, the places you touch, or the order of application. Find out whether any technique does not sound appealing and should be avoided. Demonstrate the techniques if necessary. Be flexible. If the client feels something isn't working at any time in the session, do something else.

Some clients want to respect your expertise and not get between you and your knowledge. When a client says, "Just work your magic!," you may take this as a compliment, but don't stop there. Let them know you value their input. Give the client a choice, no matter how simple. For example, "Shall we begin the session with you lying face up on the table or face down?" or "Do you prefer that work be done on your low back while you are prone or supine?" or "Should I work on your neck to release the pain you feel in your hand?" Most clients are not accustomed to being asked for their input. It may take a little encouragement for them to discover that they really do have opinions and preferences. Always give clients the option to choose how, when, and where their treatment should be applied. Make sure you give them plenty of information on which to base their decisions.

Involve your clients during the massage itself as well as during treatment planning. As you are working, invite them to notice how they feel before and after a particular technique. For example, as you move a client's shoulder, you might notice limitations in the available movement and that the quality of the movement is compromised. Rather than point out the limitations, ask what the client notices. "How does this shoulder feel to you as I move it? Now move it yourself. How does that feel?" Apply the predetermined massage technique and move the shoulder again. "Now how does your shoulder feel?" Show the client how to perform the same or similar techniques at home to get the same result. Don't make the techniques mysterious or magical. Share your expertise and knowledge and empower your clients to heal themselves.

EVALUATE PROGRESS AND PROVIDE FEEDBACK

Communicate through all stages of the interview by evaluating the client's progress and sharing feedback that can strengthen, modify, or correct the results. Progress hinges on all aspects of the therapeutic relationship: communication; trust; faith in the client's strength and healing abilities; quality of touch; understanding the client's needs; developing meaningful goals; providing education; and listening to the body, mind, and soul of the client. If you intend to give quality service, you must evaluate each step of the healing process and elicit feedback from the client continually.

Evaluate progress by summarizing your observations: what you hear, what you feel, what you see, what you interpret. You can present your summary to the client immediately after your observation, during the post-interview, or at scheduled reevaluation periods, depending on how pertinent the information is. For example, the client's response to a treatment technique may be critical if it is the first time the technique has been used or the response was significant. Otherwise, wait until the end of the session to summarize the results. At the end of a series of sessions, evaluate the massages together. Were the goals accomplished? Was the treatment style effective? Which techniques will you continue to use? Receive the feedback with an open mind and heart. Modify your treatment plan to accommodate the client's preferences.

Use assessment techniques to reinforce the results of the session. Help the client experience the changes in his body on many levels: physically, mentally, and emotionally. Often, clients leave the session with little awareness of their progress. They may feel better but have no context to understand their experience or words to explain the sensations. Verbalize your findings and demonstrate the increased movement. Have them observe postural changes in the mirror and celebrate the progress. Compliment them on their ability to respond to the treatment and to integrate changes. Help them recognize their contribution to the results and reinforce the effects their homework will have on maintaining and furthering their progress.

Regularly schedule reevaluation sessions. Some clients are shy about giving feedback during the session. They may feel vulnerable on the table or they may enter a deep state of relaxation that makes it inappropriate to push for feedback. Setting aside time periodically for evaluation can provide a safety net for clients and will let them know you are committed to hearing their concerns and responding to their needs.

SUMMARY

Developing the therapeutic relationship is central to the interview process and is even more important than gathering information or accurately assessing the client's condition. Trust, compassion, and understanding are the cornerstones of a productive relationship. Your ability to be fully present for your clients and to exhibit faith in their strength and healing abilities help lay these cornerstones in place. Without a strong bond, clients are reluctant to share their concerns, and treatment planning becomes a guessing game.

Concentrate on building the therapeutic relationship while striving to achieve the goals of the interview. Your tasks include:

1. Create a relationship.
2. Share information.
3. Develop goals for health.
4. Select and implement solutions.
5. Evaluate progress and provide feedback.

Communication is critical to achieving the goals of the interview. Employ the following verbal and nonverbal skills:

◆ Door-openers, open-ended questions
◆ Active listening: reflecting, paraphrasing, summarizing
◆ Complimenting
◆ Body language, including eye contact, posture, gestures
◆ Silence
◆ Touch

Develop and use communication skills. Lead clients to discover and accomplish goals for health. Maintain an open line of communication throughout the pre-interview, interview, hands-on interview, and post-interview. Ensure optimal results for the client by eliciting feedback with the intent to strengthen, modify, and correct the treatment plan.

REFERENCES

1. Remen RN. Kitchen Table Wisdom: Stories That Heal. New York: Riverhead Books, 1996.
2. Bolton R. People Skills: How to Assert Yourself, Listen to Others, and Resolve Conflict. New York: Simon & Schuster, 1979.
3. DeJong P, Berg IK. Interviewing for Solutions. Pacific Grove, CA: Brooks/Cole, 1998.
4. Hafen BQ, Karren KJ, Frandsen KJ, Smith NL. Mind/Body Health: The Effects of Attitudes, Emotions, and Relationships. Boston, MA: Allyn & Bacon, 1996.
5. Taylor K. The Ethics of Caring: Honoring the Web of Life in Our Professional Healing Relationships. 2nd Ed. Santa Cruz, CA: Handford Mead, 1995.
6. Carlson R, Shield B. Healers on Healing. Los Angeles, CA: Tarcher Inc., 1989.
7. Carnegie D. How to Win Friends and Influence People. New York: Pocket Books, 1936.
8. Chödrön P. Start Where You Are: A Guide to Compassionate Living. Boston, MA: Shambhala, 1994.
9. Werner R. Pathology for Massage Therapists. Baltimore, MD: Lippincott Williams & Wilkins, 1998.
10. Cherkin DC, Eisenberg D, Sherman KJ, Barlow W, Kaptchuk TJ, Street J, Deyo RA. Randomized trial comparing traditional Chinese medical acupuncture, therapeutic massage, and self-care education for chronic low back pain. Arch Intern Med 2001;161.
11. de Shazer S. The death of resistance. Family Process. 1984;23.

CHAPTER 2

*W*hy Document?

CHAPTER OUTLINE

*S*andee was a middle-aged woman with a history of chronic pain, which was becoming a way of life for her. She had tried drug therapies and even surgery to rid the agony of debilitating back pain, but it seemed to be getting worse rather than better. On the advice of a friend, Sandee began to explore massage therapy. She tried out a few therapists and started seeing Holly, a licensed massage therapist who specialized in chronic pain conditions. Holly thought things were going well, but then Sandee approached her for a referral—she wanted the name of another therapist who might better be able to rid her of pain.

Holly was familiar with this kind of frustration and told Sandee that, of course, she knew several good massage therapists in the area. She gently asked Sandee to have a seat so they could go over Sandee's file and discuss her goals and results together. Holly wanted to clearly understand Sandee's goals for health so she could adequately select a therapist to match Sandee's specific needs.

As Sandee sat down, Holly laid out 10 pages in front of her—10 pictures with Sandee's own handwriting on them. As with all her clients before each session, Holly had asked Sandee to draw the location of the pain on a page with a human figure on it. Now, seeing all the pictures together, Sandee found it impossible to deny the changes that had taken place. She could hardly take her eyes off the drawings. Her hand shook in amazement as she retraced the circles of pain she had drawn over the figure's back. On her first visit, Sandee had drawn a big circle around the entire low back and hips, a circle larger than the figure itself, and on a pain scale of one to 10 had numbered nine. Each picture that followed showed the circle of pain shrinking in size and the intensity of the pain diminishing in number. Today's figure showed a circle tightly drawn around the sacrum and marked with the number four.

Softly, Holly asked what living with chronic pain had been like over the years. Sandee explained that because she woke up every day in pain and went to bed every day in pain, she was frustrated. She felt that her condition was unchanged. She had gone from doctor to doctor, trying various treatments. Once again, she found herself repeating the same pattern of going from therapist to therapist, seeking an end to the pain. She had never experienced a cessation of pain and therefore concluded that there was no change in her condition.

Sandee had not recognized the subtle, progressive shifts in her pain. Looking at those pictures, however, she began to accept her healing and acknowledge the increase in time spent in her garden and the new-found energy to take her grandson to the park. She smiled at Holly and chose to continue care.

Wellness charting: records of client history, all treatment provided, and any additional comments regarding client preferences, practitioner findings, self-care education, and the like; also used to document wellness sessions with healthy clients

SOAP charting: acronym for Subjective, Objective, Assessment, and Plan; a process for providing a standard health care format for charting and documenting treatment sessions. Information is organized into four categories: S = data provided by the client, O = practitioner findings, A = functional outcomes and diagnoses, and P = treatment recommendations.

Introduction

Documentation is critical, necessary, and expected, but fun? Not exactly. None of us entered the hands-on healing arts because we loved paperwork. All massage therapists have stories of the client whose life was changed as a result of their work together. Our work is about relationships and interactions with people—that's what fuels our fire. Neither **Wellness charting** nor **SOAP** (Subjective, Objective, Assessment, Plan) **charting** deliver the same emotional satisfaction.

Yet, there may be a way for the paperwork to contribute to the success of those healing relationships. If so, we might be motivated to put more energy into the task.

Who Should Document?

Every massage therapist should document every massage therapy session. Yet, documentation is a skill and a habit that not all massage therapists have developed. Some massage therapists have not felt the need to document their sessions because they are not licensed health care providers. Others feel it necessary to chart only those clients who are referred by a physician or whose insurance company is reimbursing them for the sessions. At sporting events, health fairs, and in spas, charting seems cumbersome. Historically, consumers paid cash for their massage sessions and came without physician referrals, and thus massage therapists were accountable to no one but their clients. As a result, charting massage clients became less common, especially for one-time, palliative visits.

Our clients perceive us as health care providers, regardless of whether the state or insurance company does. As people are recognizing the benefits of massage, bodywork, and movement therapies, they are receiving manual therapy regularly for the treatment of physical, emotional, and spiritual ailments, as well as for wellness and preventative care. We are responsible for the health of others, and we must act accordingly. Massage therapy is a powerful healing tool, and we are to be accountable for the outcomes. Good documentation serves as a shield when a client claims wrongdoing, and it is a part of our providing safe and effective treatment. Documentation is a necessary skill to implement and to master in our practices.

Why Document?

A common misconception among massage therapists, whether or not we are seasoned paper pushers, is that we chart for someone else. We are driven by the belief that we have to document or we will not get paid; therefore, we chart only those who are insurance clients. Maybe we chart for fear of being sued, or we drum up a report from memory to maintain the referral flow when a doctor requests a client's file. On the other hand, we may be discouraged from charting because of pressure put on us by our employer. The spa manager, for example, may believe there is no time for clients to fill out an intake form or no space to store client files. Perhaps we need to chart for our clients.

Therapists have plenty of reasons not to document. Sometimes, we don't want to bother our clients with too many forms to fill out, especially when they arrive late for their appointment. Sometimes, we interpret a client's squirms during the interview to mean, "Hurry up and get me on the table," so we cut short our questioning. At other times, we rush through the assessments because we believe the only part of a session the client values is the hands-on part. Or we skip the closing interview so we don't disrupt the mood and spoil the work we've just done.

However, the reasons to chart far outweigh the reasons not to chart. To avoid medical complications, we have to begin with a health history. To ensure that we are using the most effective massage techniques, we need to track clients' responses to the various modalities we are employing. It is difficult to encourage clients to keep up their homework exercises when we can't remember what we asked them to do. And without written proof, it is difficult to convince them of their progress. For these and many other reasons, we must chart because we care about the safety of our clients and we want to provide the best possible service.

Ideally, serving our clients is the ultimate motivation for documentation. We document to gather and record information that ensures safe treatment and effective care, educates the client, and clearly states the results of the sessions so that the client acknowledges the benefits of massage.

We should maintain written records on all our clients, regardless of treatment goals or payment method. To tame the paper tiger, let's look through the eyes of the different parties invested in our documentation.

THE CLIENT

Professionalism

Some clients may consider massage therapy an "alternative," meaning riskier, or a less scientifically valid method than other, more traditional allopathic health care practices. With the integration of complementary therapies into mainstream health care, some people are seeking the care of practitioners they have never before considered. The acts of filling out health history forms, performing assessment tests, and answering questions while the practitioner takes notes can link wary clients to the familiar traditional therapies. This common thread can instill confidence and provide a professional atmosphere, reassuring the client that you are a health care specialist providing safe and effective health care, sports injury treatment, performance enhancement, or wellness care.

Trust

Massage therapy is intimate. Often, the clients remove their clothes and lie on a table with only a sheet covering them. When they are lying face down, they are not able to see us enter the room or move around, and they may feel vulnerable. Even if they don't remove their clothes, we may be touching them in places few people outside their immediate family touch. Filling out health questionnaires may provide them with a sense of confidence and a feeling that their concerns are our concerns. Interviews focused on gathering and giving information may ease their minds about how we will touch them and why. The act of taking notes demonstrates that what happens in the session is being recorded. All these things may contribute to building a solid relationship before we ever put our hands on the person. When we demonstrate concern for the client's goals for health and take a professional approach, in part through note taking, we may build a strong bond of trust that can contribute to a successful, productive relationship. The hands-on part of the session may not be the only part that has value after all.

Historical Record

A client's file is a historical record of wellness and health challenges over time, tracking health patterns and documenting massage approaches. This is a valuable resource from the client's perspective for many reasons. Clients may move or change practitioners and need to get their new massage therapists up to speed to avoid wasting time or money. Other health care providers may seek clues in our charts regarding progressive conditions—information that ultimately could help the client move toward recovery.

Safety

Clients need to feel safe in our hands. Repeatedly asking for the same information every week does not do much to instill a feeling of safety. A written record serves as a database or repository of pertinent information. In completing a thorough health history, clients are assured that the practitioner has access to information that will assist in determining safe and appropriate massage modalities for them given their goals for health. Nothing is left to memory, and clients do not have to repeat information at every session to be assured that precautions will be taken.

Proof of Progress

As in Sandee's story, it is difficult to maintain an accurate perspective of one's condition when one lives with daily pain. Having an ongoing and periodic account of one's experience and expression of health is critical to supplementing subjective memory. Daily charting can serve as a witness to the client's pain and progress.

Quality Assurance and Value

If progress is evident and goals are being met, clients may rest assured that their money is being spent well. Massage therapy is one form of health care that people have traditionally paid for out of pocket.[1] (A testament to positive outcomes!) This means we are competing with the groceries, mortgage payments, and childcare. Typically, for people to feel good about how they spend their money, the end product must outweigh the expense or the need must be based in survival. Proper documentation can express our goal-oriented approach and record the physical results, thus proving the value. Even emotional and spiritual results have a measurable physical expression. If we are not able to demonstrate long-term, positive results, we may expect our clients to seek better value for their time and money somewhere else.

Education

Documentation performed in the presence of the client can be an educational experience. The intended result is to encourage clients to participate more fully in their treatment. By participating in the documentation process, they may experience the results on a deeper level, understand what contributes to positive results, and become motivated to progress more quickly. Often, they will learn by seeing what is written down and begin to understand what is working and what is not and why, including what the plan is for the future. They know that you, their therapist, is going to hold them accountable for their homework because you wrote it down and habitually will check in with them about it. Involving clients in their massage, which includes charting, gets them participating actively and committed to their goals for health. This educational experience can instill a sense of confidence in their own ability to care for themselves and to control the way they experience their situation, which ultimately is the best outcome we can provide for our clients.

THE PRACTITIONER

Financial Security

Client files that demonstrate positive outcomes can be financially advantageous. Whether you are self-employed or are working in a clinic, client flow depends primarily on your ability to form productive, healing relationships with your clients. Successful results lead to repeat clients and solid referrals. Having documented evidence is helpful for proving your effectiveness. Documentation helps clients keep a positive perspective when they lose sight of their progress—when, for example, they can't see beyond their immediate pain—and demonstrates subjective and objective outcomes as a result of your care to referring caregivers who have greater access to your charts than to your healing hands.

Documentation is often the only evidence a health care provider (HCP) has of those successful client relationships.

Legal Assurance

In malpractice suits, your documentation can save you more than money. Malpractice suits filed against massage therapists are rare.[2] In the unfortunate event that you are named as a defendant in a malpractice case, your job and reputation may be on the line. When seeking jobs or preferred provider status, applicants may be rejected by insurance plans on the basis of complaints filed.

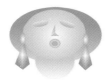

STORY TELLER
Winning and Losing

In my experience with a malpractice suit, thorough documentation showed that the symptoms the plaintiff accused my colleague's treatment of causing existed months before care was provided at my clinic. Good documentation on behalf of my colleague and the client's physicians contributed to a positive result for us.

Here is a completely different situation, one in which the lack of documentation produced a detrimental result. I received a phone call asking for support in a malpractice suit. A person had filed for damages as a result of an on-site massage at a health fair. The catch was that the person never really received a massage at the booth. However, no documentation existed to prove it: no sign-in sheet, no signed medical release form, and no treatment notes on any recipient at the booth. A favorable outcome for the massage therapist and the company that ran the booth seemed unlikely. Without written records, few opportunities exist to fight for your innocence. Protect yourself with documentation.

Professional Image

Hands-on healing has existed for thousands of years. Unfortunately, the history has shown that massage sometimes has been associated with sex for money. Perhaps no other health care profession has had to fight this kind of stigma, at least to the same degree. Other manual therapy professions have had to deal with claims of quackery because scientific evidence of curative ability was lacking. With all this working against us, it behooves us to apply certain professional practices stringently. To continue to build credibility for our health care profession, every massage therapist must document every massage session. Practitioners who do not consider their modalities "treatment" may consider the possibility that any session that has a health benefit, such as increasing circulation or reducing muscular tension, is a health care modality.

Communication With a Health Care Team

The team approach to health care relies on communication for its success. Information is rarely conveyed in person. Most communication, such as referrals and progress reports, is in written form. Other members of the team evaluate our effectiveness by reading our documentation, not by experiencing our touch or hearing client testimonials. The charts and reports must reflect the client outcomes adequately, or ongoing referrals may not ensue. Regular, brief, written communications demonstrate our professionalism and high standards, and substantiate our effectiveness. HCPs are more willing to work with massage therapists who follow familiar lines of communication. Consider this to be the least expensive form of marketing available.

Historical Record

Client charts serve as a memory database, relieving us of the responsibility to remember all the details of each case. Thus, charts free us up to think ahead rather than backwards. For example, instead of struggling to remember whether the right foot or the left foot had the broken metatarsal or whether the strain/counterstrain technique or the muscle energy technique (MET) produced the quickest result, we can simply reapply the MET to the right foot, reassess, and move on to another stage of the massage session.

Safety

A universal vow of health care providers is to do no harm. We are in this profession because we want to help others. We need to educate ourselves appropriately about our presenting clients, and we need to discover adequate information about them to assist in making safe decisions about massage. A health history can provide information about past or current illnesses and pathologies that are potentially aggravated by some modalities. We can track the client's response to massage through the daily charts and reduce the risk of overtreatment. Documentation gives us access to client information that helps us do our job with reasonable skill and safety, whether we provide wellness massage, sports massage, or clinical treatment.

Efficiency

People on the paying end of health care generally insist that the care they receive is the most effective care available for the least amount of money.[3] To be efficient in the available time, the therapist needs to know what has been effective in the past. Health history can provide information about treatments that have been used for past conditions and give insight into their effectiveness. Keep a running log of the modalities you have used and the clients' responses to them. Wellness charts or SOAP charts record treatments and track the results. This information aids in creating individualized, effective treatment plans. Each session builds on the last, for increased productivity.

SOAP charting in particular provides a system for tracking massage modalities that are effective. This information allows you to make decisions that streamline the care you are providing, on an individual and general basis. You may wish to study the results you have achieved with a given modality or for a particular condition. Reviewing many client files allows you to use your own case load as research and to evaluate your own effectiveness as a practitioner.

Clear Boundaries

Client charts may also serve as a reminder to separate your experience from that of the client. Transference and countertransference are as real in massage therapy as in psychotherapy. The line between a client's experience and the practitioner's experience can become blurred. It is not uncommon for therapists to assume the frustration of a client and mistake that feeling for their own. Use charts as a reminder of your successes and your client's accomplishments. Evaluate plateaus in the client's progress with your self-esteem intact. One helpful approach is to review the client's files before every session to establish your own feelings and prevent yourself from being drawn into the client's feelings.

THE PROFESSION

Positive Image

Massage therapy organizations are invested in the public perception of their profession. Associations provide a professional affiliation; promote education, ethics, and standards; and work as a group to provide public education and increase public awareness. These benefits are highly regarded by members and consumers alike. Documentation is often discussed, defined, and required as part of these standards.

The massage therapy profession values its relationship with the health care, spa, and sports communities. The public may view the integration of massage therapy into traditional health care as a stamp of approval that legitimizes the work. Increased public exposure at sporting events increases the number of people who become open to receiving massage therapy. The number of massage therapists entering the profession will grow as a result, and membership in professional associations will grow accordingly.

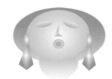

STORY TELLER
Massage Therapy at the Olympics

For the first time in our history, thanks in large part to the efforts of Benny Vaughn, massage therapists became sanctioned members of the medical team at the summer Olympic Games in Atlanta, Georgia, in 1996. At the Track and Field venue where I worked, all treatment—massage, physical therapy, and hydrotherapy—was documented as a matter of course.

Research

Research data supporting the efficacy and cost effectiveness of massage therapy validates its use as a viable treatment modality and promotes public access. No one likes to take risks with other people's health. Insurance companies and physicians rely on research results to help them make informed decisions regarding health care options. With good data, massage therapy becomes increasingly available to all who can benefit from hands-on healing. Traditional methods of research are difficult to apply to massage therapy. Case studies provide qualitative information and are a popular method of research for drugless therapies. Case study research is only as good as the therapist's documentation.

SUMMARY

Massage therapists who practice effective documentation display professionalism and high standards, and they ensure client safety in all massage environments, whether in sports arenas, spas, or on-site locations. In clinical practices, charting assists massage therapists in communicating easily with other health care professionals. Documentation is vital to case study research, which provides statistics supporting health care integration and increased public access.

Massage therapists benefit in a variety of ways when they document client relationships. It makes good business sense to protect our investment of time and services by charting the client's condition, the necessity of care, and the effectiveness of the treatment provided. Adequate documentation can help us avoid potential legal difficulties. Client charts can be used as a communication tool with health care providers—to provide evidence of client progress and the effectiveness of massage—and to encourage future referrals. Communication through documentation establishes rapport within the health care team, promotes a team approach to treatment, and ensures that clients have been cared for effectively when transition is necessary.

Our clients also benefit from our documentation efforts. In their eyes, thorough charting demonstrates our professionalism and high standards, provides written proof of their own progress and the value of their time and resources, documents the efficacy of our treatment so they can feel confident about their decision to receive massage therapy, and provides an awareness that they can contribute to a higher quality of life for themselves.

REFERENCES

1. Eisenberg D, Kessler RC, Foster C, et al. Unconventional medicine in the United States: Prevalence, costs, and patterns of use. N Engl J Med 1993;328.
2. Sperger M. Interview of Marlys Sperger, Executive Director of the American Massage Therapy Association, 2000.
3. HMO Washington Participating Health Care Provider Agreement, 1996.

after getting persciption after 1st massage

1. Righe and intione report and intedotin

2. send Sope notes

3. ounght for progret repont need more time or have met goles

CHAPTER **3**

_D_ocumentation: Intake Forms

CHAPTER OUTLINE

David was a good student. He performed his duties in student clinic professionally and sincerely. One day, after a 30-minute massage on an elderly client's neck and shoulders, the client looked up suddenly and said, "I forgot to tell you, I have blood clots in my neck." As David learned early in school, thrombosis is a contraindication for massage—blood clots could become dislodged and move toward the brain, resulting in a stroke. Luckily, the woman was not harmed by the session, and David learned a poignant lesson in the importance of taking a thorough health history.

Introduction

Intake forms are the first step in gathering information from the client. They provide general questions about personal identification, contact information, health history, and current goals for health. This chapter introduces a variety of intake forms, including:

◆ Health information form
◆ Fee schedule and policies form
◆ Health report form

All these forms are completed before the initial session. The health information form is updated annually, and the health report form may be completed periodically to evaluate progress or be filled out before and after every session as an elementary form of charting. The fee schedule and policies form is distributed at the initial session and updated as needed. This chapter explains the purpose of each form and provides assistance in determining its appropriate application for your practice and for each client.

Intake forms are easy to use and don't require one-on-one attention from the massage therapist. They are self-explanatory and can be filled out by the client before the initial session, without cutting into precious treatment time. It is a good idea to go over the forms with the client after they have been completed to ensure that they are filled out accurately and to add pertinent details.

Once you have reviewed the forms, you are well-equipped to ask specific, personalized questions based on the information provided. These in-depth interviews are important in developing a better understanding of the individuals with whom you are working and their unique concerns and goals for health. Think of the forms and the ensuing interviews as stepping stones to building healing relationships.

Personalize your intake forms with your logo and business information. Space is provided at the top of each form (see Figure 3-1). Your name, address, and phone number should be imprinted on every page in the client's chart. This is to ensure that you have identification in the event that your charts become part of an **audit** or **subpoena** or the client shares his or her file with another health care provider or therapist. An easy and inexpensive solution is to have a rubber stamp made of your contact information. Place your stamp in a position on the page where you won't lose information if your filing system requires holes to be punched at the top of your forms.

Health Information Forms: For Wellness Massage

A variety of brief health information forms have been adapted specifically for relaxation massage, spa therapies, on-site massage, or sports massage. Many clients use massage therapy to stay

audit: a formal and often periodic examination of accounts, financial records, or claims to verify correctness of documentation (An internal peer review process has been used to evaluate the quality of care provided and assess medical necessity.)

subpoena: court-ordered, written command requiring a person to appear at a specific time and place to give testimony on a specific matter. A *subpoena duces tecum* is a written command requiring a witness to produce documents in his or her possession or control that are pertinent to the issues.

healthy and reduce stress. Others strive for ease and efficiency while performing athletic and artistic activities. Massage therapy can be used to refine skills they already have or help them enjoy being active late in life. Intake questions that address these goals for health are designed to be quick and easy to use and to ensure the safety of the patient. Less emphasis is placed on gathering a comprehensive list of symptoms and specific facts regarding the client's medical condition that may be superfluous to wellness massage (see Figure 3-2).

The health information form on the Wellness chart meets the three basic needs for alternative documentation:

◆ It is quick and easy to use.
◆ It helps ensure the clients' safety.
◆ It assists in providing legal protection for the practitioner.

QUICK AND EASY CHARTING

The Wellness intake questions indicate yes or no answers that can be checked off quickly by the client. In an on-site or sports venue, the questions can be asked orally and only positive answers are recorded by the massage therapist. When reading the intake questions aloud, make eye contact to ensure that the client is paying attention and has an understanding of the questions being asked. The questions are brief but critical. For example, at a sporting event, the form may help determine whether first aid is more appropriate than massage.

CLIENT SAFETY

Intake questions are designed to ensure the safety of the client. Wellness charts have very few intake questions, but the questions are designed to get right to health issues. Any yes answer to an intake question can require additional information to rule out potential harm. The massage therapist must be able to identify health situations that contraindicate treatment or require precautionary measures before treatment is provided. For example,

---

FIGURE 3-1 Wellness Health Information—Personalized Header Sample

Naomi Wachtel
567 Sunnydale Dr.
Flat Irons, CO   80302
TEL   303 555 8866   **WELLNESS CHART**

Name _Lin Pak_____ ID#/DOB _5-31-63_____ Date _7-27-04_____
Phone __(303) 555-0033 x 253_____ Address __IBM 3rd Floor_____

1. What are your goals for health, and how may I assist you in achieving your goals? _Limit_____
    longterm complications of diabetes through relaxation and stress reduction.

2. List typical daily activities—work, exercise, home. _I sit a lot at work and watch movies_____
    at home

3. Are you currently experiencing any of the following? If yes, please explain.
    pain, tenderness   ☒ No ☐ Yes: _____   stiffness ☒ No ☐ Yes: _____

inflammation may indicate infection, which contraindicates circulatory massage. Numbness contraindicates deep pressure. Some symptoms contraindicate locally but not systemically, and some techniques are contraindicated but not others.[1] Learn how to respond to positive answers to intake questions. Refer to Werner's *A Massage Therapist's Guide to Pathology*, published by Lippincott Williams & Wilkins (2002), for more information on contraindications and precautions for massage therapy.

Adapt the intake questions to discover possible contraindications specific to your work environment. For example, the intake questions for a sporting event cover signs and symptoms of shock—the primary contraindication for treatment after physical stress. Intake questions for a spa environment emphasize allergies to scents, oils, and other products used during aromatherapy and herbal wraps. Include information-gathering questions specific to the treatment provided, such as whether or not the client has an allergy to honey.

LEGAL PROTECTION

Protect yourself in the rare event of a malpractice case by demonstrating that health screening was considered and treatment was appropriate. To do this, have the client fill out, sign, and date a health questionnaire. If you complete the form for the client, require the client to initial the entries. Show that you checked for possible health complications and provided safe treatment.

FIGURE 3-2 Sports Chart—Intake Questions Sample

WELLNESS CHART—SPORTS

Massage Therapist _Naomi Wachtel, LMT_ Date _7-4-04_

Event _Mountain Aid 10K_   Location _Finish Line Tent_

Ask each athlete the following: (Note individual responses below—concerns only.)

1. Are you currently experiencing any of the following?
   - pain, tenderness, stiffness   • swelling
   - numbness, tingling   • dizziness
   - cold, clammy skin   • shaking

2. How soon do you compete? / When did you finish competing?

3. Have you warmed up? / Cooled down?

4. Have you consumed water since the event?

Athlete's Name _Janelle Helm_   Athlete's initials: _JH_

Hx: (note concerns) _No water – gave her 12 oz before Tx_

Tx: (check all that apply) _____ Pre-event ✓ _____ Post-event _____ Refer-first aid/med

C: _gave her 12 oz after Tx_   Initials: _NW_

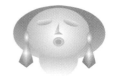

Always look over the health history before proceeding with the treatment. A malpractice case was filed accusing an on-site massage therapist of harming a client. Before the session, the therapist handed the intake form to the client. The client read the form and handed it back to the practitioner without completing it. The massage therapist proceeded with the treatment without realizing that the client had not signed off on the statement of health. As it turned out, the person had one of the conditions listed as a contraindication on the form and alleged he was injured as a result of the treatment provided. Take steps to protect yourself and follow through with them.

Health Information Form: For Treatment Massage

CONTENT

A comprehensive health information form designed for clients with medical conditions, such as whiplash, sports injuries, or carpel tunnel syndrome, records five basic kinds of information:

- Personal identification and contact information
- Current health information
- Goals for health
- History of injuries, illnesses, and surgeries
- Contract for care

(See Appendix: Blank Forms)

Personal Identification and Contact Information

The client's name, date of birth or insurance identification number, and the date the form is completed should appear on every piece of paper in the client's file. The name connects the data to a living, breathing person and can be used to organize the files. Date of birth differentiates individuals who have the same name—for clients seeking insurance reimbursement for massage sessions, use their insurance identification number instead. An insurance identification number can be used for the same purpose as the date of birth and will assist clients in obtaining reimbursement. The date places the information in time, an important reference for tracking the progress of the condition. When multiple entries are made on a single page, each entry should be dated.

Record all possible contact numbers on the health information form. Know how to reach clients in a timely fashion in case appointments need to be changed or issues need to be discussed. Always protect their confidentiality and do not disclose details of the appointment or treatment, such as by leaving a detailed message on a phone system without permission to do so.

In the unlikely event of an emergency, be prepared. Have each client list a contact person who can be reached immediately in case of a sudden illness or accident. On the health information form, request the permission of your client to consult with other health care providers on the client's team (see Figure 3-3). This request is courteous, and it models

45

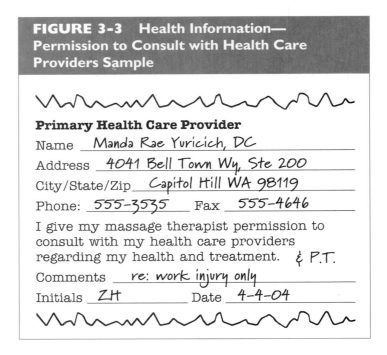

FIGURE 3-3 Health Information—Permission to Consult with Health Care Providers Sample

Primary Health Care Provider

Name _Manda Rae Yuricich, DC_

Address _4041 Bell Town Wy, Ste 200_

City/State/Zip _Capitol Hill WA 98119_

Phone: _555-3535_ Fax _555-4646_

I give my massage therapist permission to consult with my health care providers regarding my health and treatment. _& P.T._

Comments _re: work injury only_

Initials _ZH_ Date _4-4-04_

open communication. Most clients assume you will be in touch with their referring HCP. Others will appreciate being asked. Even if clients were not referred by an HCP, they may have a condition that warrants a consultation with their primary HCP. Their doctors may not know they are receiving massage therapy, and they may want the chance to tell their doctors first. Some clients may share information with you that they don't want discussed with others. Let them know the information you plan to share, with whom and why. This simple permission request is sufficient for most purposes. If you are required to comply with the **Health Insurance Portability and Accountability Act (HIPAA)** regarding confidentiality because you store and transfer client data electronically, use a HIPAA-approved consent form in addition to this health information form. (For more information regarding HIPAA compliance, visit http://www.aspe.hhs.gov/admnsimp/index.shtml.)

Health care providers are exempt if they do not submit electronic claims, if no billing company or other third party on behalf of the care provider transmits any such information electronically, and if they do not accept Medicare.

Health Insurance Portability and Accountability Act (HIPAA): federal regulation intended to improve the effectiveness and efficiency of the health care system by standardizing the electronic transmission of health information and protect the security and privacy of health information

Current Health Information

In this section of the form, clients are asked to list, prioritize, and classify current health concerns and identify the way (or ways) in which those conditions are affecting daily life (see Figure 3-4). The goal is to discover why individual clients are seeking treatment, so you can address their needs and contribute to their goals for health. Specific questions help clients clarify their reasons for seeking massage therapy. Unmet expectations are often the product of unspoken desires. Leave little room for interpretation and be clear about clients' goals for the massage therapy sessions.

In addition to being a record of clients' concerns, this form provides questions about treatments clients have received for these conditions in the past and any self-care strategies they have practiced. Use this information to formulate a treatment plan. Eliminate techniques that were ineffective, avoid those that other practitioners on the health care team are using, and incorporate or encourage solutions the client has found helpful. Consider your clients' goals for the session and together, with your ideas for a treatment approach, discuss the various options in the interview.

FIGURE 3-4 Health Information—Current Health Information Sample

B. Current Health Information

List Health Concerns Check all that apply

Primary ___back pain___
- ☐ mild ☒ moderate ☐ disabling
- ☒ constant ☐ intermittant
- ☒ symptoms ↑ w/activity   ☐ ↓ w/activity
- ☒ getting worse ☐ getting better ☐ no change
treatment received ___pain pills, back brace___

Secondary ___headaches___
- ☐ mild ☒ moderate ☐ disabling
- ☐ constant ☒ intermittant
- ☒ symptoms ↑ w/activity   ☐ ↓ w/activity
- ☒ getting worse ☐ getting better ☐ no change
treatment received ___pain pills___

Additional ___neck stiff___
- ☒ mild ☐ moderate ☐ disabling
- ☒ constant ☐ intermittant
- ☒ symptoms ↑ w/activity   ☐ ↓ w/activity
- ☐ getting worse ☒ getting better ☐ no change
treatment received ___stretching___

List Daily Activities Limited by Condition

Work ___N/A___

Home/Family ___gardening, vacuuming___

Sleep/Self-care ___sleep, exercise___

Social/Recreational ___play w/ grandchildren,___
___dancing, bowling, bridge group___

List Self-Care Routines

How do you reduce stress? ___watch sports,___
___garden___
Pain? ___heat, back brace, meds___

List current medications (include pain relievers and herbal remedies) _____
___hydrocodone 500 mg every 4 hrs___

Have you ever received massage therapy before? ___no___ Frequency? _____

What are your goals for receiving massage therapy? ___get around easier, less pain___

If the client's condition is recent and he or she has not yet received treatment, look to the general health history for information regarding a treatment approach. Something in your client's history may have contributed to his current health, or the treatment sought for other conditions may provide information that could shape a successful treatment plan for the unique individual before you. You can get a sense of the client's preferences in treatment based on the type of self-care he or she has incorporated into a daily routine: conventional or alternative; participatory or passive.

Health History

This section consists of two parts: (1) a chart listing surgeries, accidents, and major illnesses; and (2) a checklist of symptoms and conditions. The chart allows clients to identify major health crises and provides quick referencing for the practitioner. This information can provide insight into the origin of current conditions or identify factors that may influence those conditions (see Figure 3-5).

FIGURE 3-5 Health Information—Health History Sample

C. Health History

List and Explain. Include dates and treatment received.

Surgeries   _none_

Injuries   _Broken arm ⓡ fell out of tree house in 1987, cast for 8 wks_

Major Illnesses   _none_

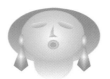

STORY TELLER
Health History Affects Current Condition

Physical trauma can result in weakness and compensational posture or movement patterns, especially when untreated. These complications may cause concomitant dysfunction or may contribute to chronic conditions. In one of our staff meetings, we discovered that the majority of clients with chronic repetitive stress injuries treated at the clinic had a history of previous soft tissue trauma, with whiplash topping the list. Sara, for example, was in a car accident as a teenager. She bounced right back and never thought about the experience again. Twenty years later, she suffers from recurring thoracic outlet syndrome. A pattern was emerging: In the winter, she painted every wall and ceiling in her house; in the summer, she refinished the hardwood floors, and every spring after long gardening sprees, she came to the clinic complaining of numbness and tingling in her right arm and hand. It wasn't until we discussed her case as a group that we considered her past history. The accident was so long ago that no one gave it much thought. Once we determined that Sara had a poorly healed cervical sprain-strain injury, her treatment plan shifted and her recurring condition subsided. Sara's case demonstrates that the chronological chart can help you identify pre-existing conditions that are adversely affecting current conditions. This prompts you to adjust the treatment plan to address the old trauma.

Following the chart is a checklist of symptoms and conditions, organized by body systems. The checklist provides an easy way to identify other factors that may be contributing to the current symptoms and to pinpoint conditions that may require special precautions. You can then apply your knowledge of indications and contraindications to the development of your treatment plan (see Figure 3-6).

FIGURE 3-6 Health Information—Checklist Sample

General

current	past		comments
☒	☐	headaches	MVA
☒	☒	pain	scoliosis
☒	☐	sleep disturbances	
			can't get comfortable
☐	☒	fatigue	scoliosis
☐	☐	infections	
☐	☐	fever	
☐	☐	sinus	
☐	☐	other	

Contract and Consent for Care

The contract for care is an invitation for the client to participate in treatment and to share the responsibility for the result. It delineates the client's commitment to the healing relationship. The goal is to empower the client to become active in the healing process and to promise goodwill on behalf of the massage therapist.

The consent for care states that the client is actively choosing massage therapy and giving permission to the practitioner to provide treatment. It may warn of possible risks and limitations of the therapy. Know the limits of your **scope of practice** and state them clearly here. Include a statement about your practice philosophy and how you intend to assist the client toward greater health.

scope of practice: law defining the standards of competence, practice areas, and conduct of a health care provider

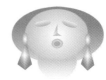

STORY TELLER
Sample Scope of Practice and Treatment Statement

As a licensed massage therapist, George uses this scope of practice statement in Washington, a state with a legally defined scope:

"I understand that massage therapists do not diagnose medical, physical, or mental disorders, nor do they perform spinal manipulations by the use of a thrusting force. I acknowledge that massage therapy is not a substitute for medical examinations or treatment; massage therapy is complementary to medical services."

George explains the intent of his treatment sessions on his health information form this way:

"Massage therapy is intended to help you learn more about the dynamics of health that are within your control—increased awareness of your patterns of movement and holding, responses to stress, and accumulation of tension. Massage therapy is a holistic approach to bridging mind and body. Together we will recognize your physical signals of diminishing health and enable you to respond to them in ways that promote vitality, balance, and spirit."

End the health information form with a dated signature confirming that the information provided is complete and accurate and that the client is consenting to treatment. If the client is under age 18, require the signature of a parent or legal guardian. This signed statement is sometimes referred to as a treatment disclaimer or waiver. The client's signature on the form may not legally protect you if something goes awry, but it demonstrates informed decision making regarding safe care. However, the most important element of the contract and consent for care is the verbal discussion that leads to an agreement to engage in a therapeutic relationship. As Jerry A. Green, a malpractice attorney in California and president of the Medical Decision Making Institute, states, "Remember: Legal problems begin as disagreements. You prevent legal problems by making meaningful agreements."[2]

TIMING AND APPLICATION

A thorough history takes time to recreate. Instruct the client to arrive 15 to 30 minutes before the initial appointment to ensure adequate time for filling out the forms. You may choose to save time by mailing out the health information form and all other applicable intake forms to the client a week before the first session. People may breeze through the forms in your office because they are eager to get on with the session. When given their own time to think about the questions, to look up things if necessary, or to ask family members for help in reconstructing events, their information tends to be more complete. Occasionally, people forget to bring the forms to the initial session, but most of them remember and mail the forms in advance. Even if they forget the forms, filling them out a second time goes much more quickly.

Regardless of individual goals for massage, each client should complete a basic health information form annually. Whenever the client has progressive or degenerative health problems or when the client's health changes, the form should be updated semiannually or quarterly.

Use the form as an information database and refer to it for interviewing the client, designing the treatment plan, identifying possible cautions for care, and contacting the client throughout the relationship.

Fees and Policies
CONTENT

Publish your fees and policies and distribute them to all clients. Determine the policies that allow you to be financially sound and provide clear boundaries to clients. You can always be more lenient later (if special circumstances arise), but it is difficult to get tough after the fact. Ensure your safety by defining the client behavior necessary for you to relax and enjoy your practice.

fee schedules: maximum allowable charges; amounts set by the insurer as the highest amounts to be charged for particular services

Current Procedural Terminology (CPT) codes: listing of descriptive terms and identifying codes for reporting health care services and procedures performed by health care providers

Fee Schedules

Fee schedules state the various services you offer and the costs associated with them. Fees may be delineated by style or intent, such as wellness or treatment massage; by modalities, such as Manual Lymphatic Drainage or Feldenkrais; or by service codes, such as Massage Therapy–97124 or Manual Therapy–97140 (see Figure 3-7).

Define each service clearly. For example, the **Current Procedural Terminology (CPT)** code book (published by the American Medical Association) defines all health care services

FIGURE 3-7 Fees and Policies—Fee Schedule Sample

A. Fee Schedule

Fees for services are as follows:

- CranioSacral/Lymph Drainage $100 per hour
  (97140)   ($25 per 15 minute unit)
- Feldenkrais $100 per hour
  (97112)   ($25 per 15 minute unit)
- Hot and Cold Packs $15 per session
  (97010)   ($15 per session)
- Therapeutic Massage $80 Per Hour
  (97124)   ($20 per 15 minute unit)

by categorizing like modalities: Massage Therapy—97124—is defined as massage, including effluerage, petrissage, and tapotement (such as stroking, compression, or percussion).[3] The purpose of the terminology is to provide a uniform language that will describe health care services accurately and will be an effective means for reliable, nationwide communication among providers, patients, and third parties. However, there is no standard terminology defining a style of massage: wellness, treatment, therapeutic, or medical. If you choose to delineate different fees for these "styles" of massage, do so with a clear definition and make sure that the specific modalities used do not overlap.

Another method for setting your fee schedule is to charge by time rather than by modalities. A flat fee is established to pay for all health care services performed under the single code. This method is known as **bundling** services. Determine a set fee that includes any massage therapy applied. For example, you may use Swedish massage, myofascial release, lymph drainage, trigger point therapy, acupressure, and muscle energy techniques in varying combinations if you find it difficult to break them down into time per modality. You can choose to define your services using the general massage therapy procedural code—97124—and not bother with four different procedure codes and four different rates. Bundling services is common in cash practices and can be used with a billing practice as long as you are not bundling procedures that would be reimbursed at a lower rate than the one under which you are billing. This practice is known as **upcoding**.

bundling: type of reimbursement arrangement that combines two or more health care procedures into one procedure code

upcoding: process of increasing a CPT code from one of lower value to one of higher value that results in a higher reimbursement rate

Office Policies

Provide written statements of your office policies. Make sure your clients read them and agree to abide by them. Require a signature demonstrating that clients have read and understand your policies. It is easier to enforce something that is written down, signed, and dated. Keep the signed form in their file. You may have to remind your clients of these policies at a later date.

Cancellation policies are common in practices in which one session makes up a significant percentage of the daily income. Set a standard cancellation fee or charge the full price of the session if the client fails to cancel within a specified number of hours before the scheduled time. Consider abiding by your own cancellation policy. For example, offer a similar discount to those clients whose appointments you cancel without a 24-hour notice, or a "free pass" for a late cancellation in the future.

Right of refusal is another common office policy. This policy can be helpful for turning away people who are impaired by alcohol or drugs, have an infectious illness, push for treatment outside your scope of practice, or behave inappropriately. It is important to set boundaries, feel safe in your practice, and have permission to take care of yourself. Use this policy any time you have a gut instinct to do so.

There may be other policies you would like to implement to enhance operations. Consider issues that might arise around parking, late arrivals, or perhaps a client giving his appointment to a friend—anything that could distract you from providing quality care. Review and update your fees and policies annually.

TIMING AND APPLICATION

The client should read and sign your fees and policies before the first session. Include the policy statement with the health information form and any other intake forms completed by the client at the initial visit. Post your fees and policies—to reinforce what you are requiring the clients to read and sign and to demonstrate your professionalism toward potential clients who walk in off the street.

Health Report
CONTENT

The health report provides a snapshot of the client's health (blank forms may be found in the Appendix: Blank Forms). In a few minutes, the client can chart the location of pain, stiffness, and numbness by writing letters—P for pain, S for stiffness, N for numbness—on illustrations of human figures and can rate his or her pain and loss of function by placing a dash on the lines of the analog scales. The drawings provide a map of the client's symptoms that is accurate and easy to read. Below the figures are two analog scales or lines of continuum: one denotes pain; the other activity level. The mark on the line is measured and a numerical score is calculated and recorded, making references to progress a snap.

The health report is the form mentioned in the case study of Sandee in Chapter 2. The benefits of this form are great for the client and the practitioner. Progress is recorded in the client's own handwriting, convincing even the most frustrated client of his or her health improvements. The massage therapist can use this form (see p. 133) to support the health history interview, gathering pertinent information from tentative clients and streamlining the discussion with the chatty ones

Human Figures

Diverse learning styles are widely employed in today's classrooms. Visual, auditory, and tactile learners have different ways of processing and storing information. The same is true for clients. Some enjoy filling out forms, others would rather tell you about themselves—and often do so in story format. Still others can draw images more easily than filling in the blanks or talking. Provide a variety of ways to gather information: multiple choice forms, one-on-one communication, and pictures to draw on, such as the ones on the health report (see Figure 3-8).

Coaxing information from some clients can feel like pulling teeth. Maybe they were taught not to complain, or they are just not comfortable speaking to people they do not know well. For those clients, drawing symptoms on pictures may be easier than having to talk about their pain or disability.

FIGURE 3-8 Health Report—Human Figures Sample

A. Draw today's symptoms on the figures.

1. Identify CURRENT symptomatic areas in your body by marking letters on the figures below. Use the letters provided in the key to identify the symptoms you are feeling today.
2. Circle the area around each letter, representing the size and shape of each symptom location.

Key
P = pain or tenderness
S = joint or muscle stiffness
N = numbness or tingling

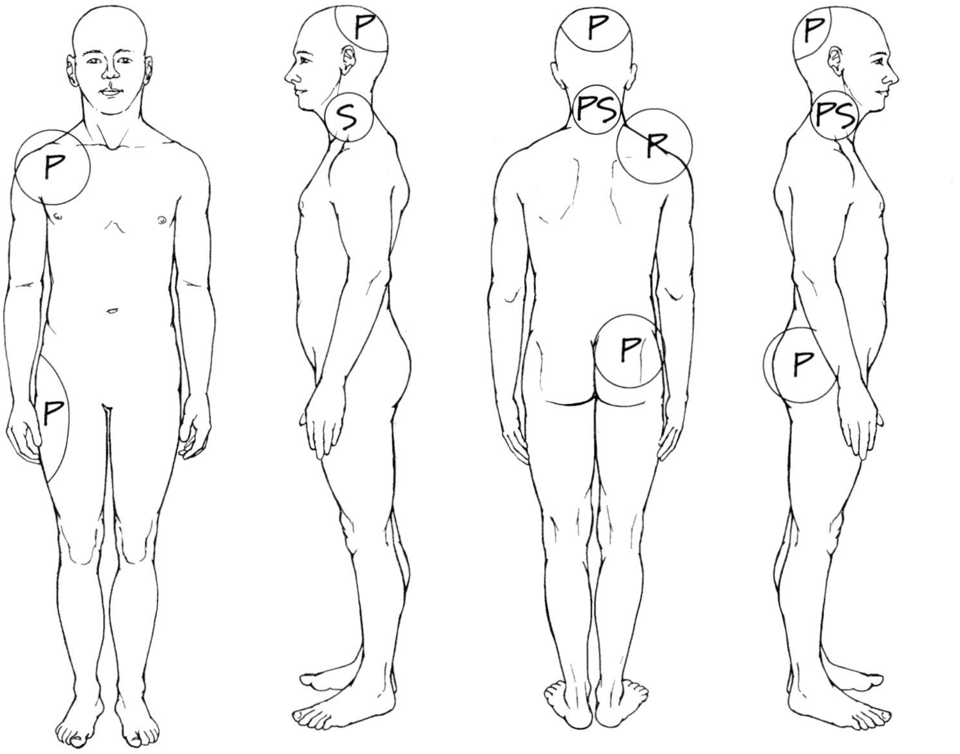

With other clients, trying to keep the interview under five minutes is challenging. Some would rather talk about their problems than solve them. Others chatter when they get nervous. Gather the salient information on a form at each session. Once the current information is recorded and reviewed, a few brief questions may suffice to prepare for the session.

Analog Scales

An analog scale is a method of measurement that uses a line of continuum and places one extreme on one end and the opposite extreme on the other end. For example, on this form (see Figure 3-9) the therapist measures her clients' pain or loss of function. On the line of continuum, pain-free is at one end and debilitating pain is at the other end. Clients place a mark at a point between the two extremes that best represents how they feel at the moment.

Analog scales are reliable and more accurate than numerical rating scales of 0 to 10. The literature suggests that numbers can be remembered from session to session, decreasing the validity of the responses. A malingerer may remember a previous response and manipulate the answer accordingly.[4]

It is cumbersome to use these scales with each subjective complaint or objective finding. A verbal response is indicated during the session; pulling out a piece of paper and a pen is inappropriate. The number scale (0 to 10) or word values (mild, moderate, severe) are preferred. Used on the health report, the analog scale is effective and addresses the two primary concerns in health care outcomes: function and pain.

To use the analog scale, the client simply places a mark on the lines to indicate pain level at that moment. The line represents a continuum ranging from pain free to unbearable pain, or from full activity to no activity. The line is 10 centimeters long, making it easy to score the client's mark on a scale of 0 to 10. On a scale of pain free to unbearable pain, for example, pain free is given the value zero, and unbearable pain is given the value ten. The mark is placed between the two values, and the measurement is assigned a value of 0 to 10. The measurement is the score. After the session, the practitioner measures the mark on the line and records the score in the comments section.

TIMING AND APPLICATION

Clients with injuries or chronic conditions should complete the health report every 30 days. If a client has no subjective complaints, such as pain, loss of function, stiff joints, or neuropathies, simply include the report in the packet of intake forms at the initial visit and the annual updates to ensure that you have all the health information you need.

The health report provides a quick and easy update on how the client is feeling at each evaulation session. Over time, it demonstrates the progress of the client and the success of the massage treatment. Thirty-day evaluations are standard protocol in health care. If either you or your client are updating the HCP on the effects of massage, you are expected to provide a report every 30 days. Make a point to evaluate the client's progress regularly, even if the client is self-referred. The client will find the updates useful. If motivating yourself to chart is an issue, this form is a simple way to ease into the habit of regular documentation. Have the client do most of the charting for you! When used before and after each session, charting records the client's presenting symptoms and the results of the session. This shortcut is not recommended for insurance clients or for long-term care, but it is a good way to get started. For use in this way, create a double-sided form with the health report on both sides. Ask the client to fill out the front of the form (Side A) before the session and the back (Side B) after the session. Use the Comments section of the form

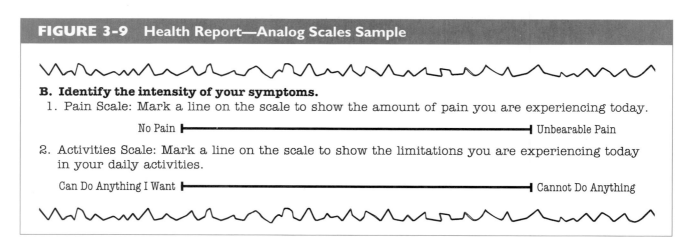

FIGURE 3-9   Health Report—Analog Scales Sample

B. Identify the intensity of your symptoms.
1. Pain Scale: Mark a line on the scale to show the amount of pain you are experiencing today.

No Pain ┣━━━━━━━━━━━━━━━━━━━━━━━━━━━━━━━━┫ Unbearable Pain

2. Activities Scale: Mark a line on the scale to show the limitations you are experiencing today in your daily activities.

Can Do Anything I Want ┣━━━━━━━━━━━━━━━━━━━━━━━━━━┫ Cannot Do Anything

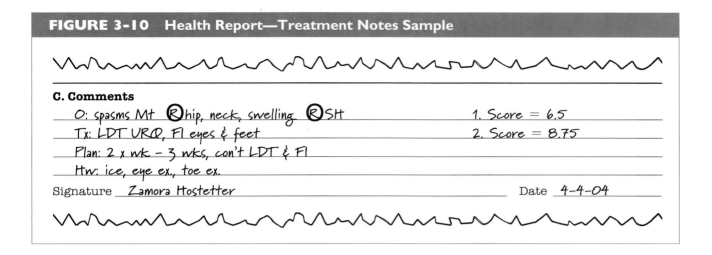

FIGURE 3-10 Health Report—Treatment Notes Sample

C. Comments

O: spasms Mt ⓇHip, neck, swelling ⓇSH   1. Score = 6.5

Tx: LDT URⓆ, Fl eyes & feet   2. Score = 8.75

Plan: 2 x wk – 3 wks, con't LDT & Fl

Hw: ice, eye ex., toe ex.

Signature *Zamora Hostetter*   Date *4-4-04*

---

to record your objective data and treatment notes. This way, the client does the presession and postsession subjective documentation for you. As you proceed through this book, you will discover the limitations of using this form for all your daily charting needs, but when necessary, begin with the health report for your daily notetaking (see Figure 3-10).

Amending the Forms

Occasionally, you may want to make slight changes, additions, or corrections to the information recorded on any of the forms in the client's file (without asking the client to complete an entirely new form). The client's perspective may change or he or she may wish to include new perceptions. Changes can be made by either the client or the practitioner, regardless of whoever originally filled out the form.

Here are two options for updating the existing form:

1. Write the new information on the original form. If you are replacing existing information, draw a single line through the outdated information, making sure that the previous information is still legible. Date and initial all changes and additions. Never white-out or erase any content or discard any information (see Figure 3-11).

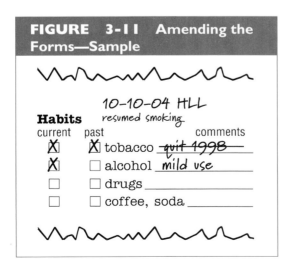

FIGURE 3-11 Amending the Forms—Sample

		10-10-04 HLL
Habits		resumed smoking
current	past	comments
☒	☒ tobacco	~~quit 1998~~
☒	☐ alcohol	*mild use*
☐	☐ drugs	
☐	☐ coffee, soda	

2. Attach an amendment to the document. Write the new information on a separate sheet of paper and staple it to the original. Date and initial the attachment.

All medical documents may be amended or updated as needed. Clients have a right to access their files and make sure the information recorded is accurate. Make a habit of recordkeeping in the presence of the client. Avoid misinformation and misinterpretations. Reiterate the information provided to you and confirm your interpretation of the client's history and current status verbally.

SUMMARY

A variety of intake forms are used to document the therapeutic relationship. All of these forms are completed before the first treatment, and some are completed periodically to evaluate progress.

Every client fills out a health information form and reads and signs a fee schedule and office policies. Clients who have health concerns and are seeking treatment for injuries or illnesses fill out a health report periodically to document subjective data and to assist the massage therapist in evaluating progress.

REFERENCES

1. Werner R. A Massage Therapist's Guide to Pathology, 2nd Ed. Baltimore, MD: Lippincott Williams & Wilkins, 2002.
2. Green JA. Holistic Practice Forum, HP–100, Green, Mill Valley, 1990.
3. AMA. CPT 2004 Standard Edition.
4. Adler RH, Giersch P. Whiplash, Spinal Trauma, and the Chiropractic Personal Injury Case. Seattle: AdlerGiersch PS, 2000.

CHAPTER 4

Wellness Charting for Sports and On-Site Massage, Relaxation and Spa Therapies, and Energy Work

CHAPTER OUTLINE

*J*ose received massage therapy weekly at the Healing Arts Clinic. He never mentioned to his massage therapists, Annie and Jamie, that he had been in a car collision. It wasn't a secret; he just didn't remember either of them asking. Jose was sure his car insurance would not cover massage because his doctor wouldn't prescribe it. Jose knew he needed something to loosen up his tense muscles and decided to pay cash for his weekly massage therapy.

Jose responded well to his massages. Annie combined Swedish techniques with deep tissue massage and gymnastics to increase mobility, loosen tight muscles, and help Jose relax. Jamie, who specialized in sports massage, used circulatory and drainage techniques. Jose found he had more energy and felt more relaxed. He believed massage was helping him recover from his car collision.

A year into his weekly massage routine, after prompting from his attorney, Jose asked the receptionist at the Healing Arts Clinic for copies of his massage records. His attorney wanted to include the massage records and bills in the settlement package for his personal injury lawsuit. The attorney intended to use the records to substantiate Jose's injuries—thereby strengthening the lawsuit—and planned to submit the bills as proof of out-of-pocket expenses Jose had incurred as a direct result of the collision. Jose had not specified any health complications and had not been referred by a doctor; and because no insurance company was paying for the sessions, Annie had chosen not to document any of the sessions. Jamie did not chart her sessions either. The receptionist had no records on Jose except cash receipts. Jose's lawyer was unable to establish a connection between the massage sessions and the injuries from the car collision without documentation. Therefore, Jose was unable to get reimbursed for the thousands of dollars he spent on massage, even though the therapy was instrumental in his recovery.

One afternoon, Jamie and Annie were sipping herbal tea at the Sunny Cafe downstairs and commiserating over their misfortune in losing their steady client, Jose. Jamie told a similar story: Claire had been a client for many years, coming monthly for relaxation massage. Then, three months ago, Claire had been injured at work. Claire's insurance company was refusing to pay for her massage therapy. The insurance adjuster claimed that because Claire had been seeing a massage therapist before the injury, she must have had pre-existing conditions that required her to continue receiving massage treatments. Therefore, the massage therapy was not necessary for treating the recent injury.

Claire had asked Jamie for her records so that she could prove to the insurance company that she had been in excellent health until the injury. Jamie had no records of the massage sessions. Even though Claire had been healthy and had received massage for relaxation only, there was no documentation to prove that to the insurance company. Claire was stuck with the bills.

Jamie and Annie shook their heads in dismay. Initially, they had been under the impression that only insurance-paying clients required documentation. Gone were the days when relaxation therapy was an excuse not to do paperwork. They made a pact with each other to better serve their clients and themselves by charting all sessions. It no longer mattered whether the session was for relaxation or injury treatment or whether payment came from an insurance company or from the client; they were going to keep records on every client and document every session.

Introduction

SOAP charting assists practitioners in solving clients' medical problems. Yet, not everyone seeks massage therapy to treat an injury or to care for an illness. Often, people in good health receive massage therapies for any number of reasons, such as relaxing and reducing stress, receiving healthy touch, or detoxifying and toning the skin.

SOAP charting: acronym for Subjective, Objective, Assessment, and Plan; a process for providing a standard health care format for charting and documenting treatment sessions. Information is organized into four categories: S = data provided by the client, O = practitioner findings, A = functional outcomes and diagnoses, and P = treatment recommendations.

If SOAP (Subjective, Objective, Assessment, Plan) charting is used to help assess, treat, and cure medical problems and the client has no pre-existing conditions or current complaints, is the practitioner obligated to keep a medical record?

Yes. Massage therapy is considered a health care modality, and practitioners are licensed, certified, or regulated in varying capacities throughout the United States and other countries. If you are practicing massage in a state or province that does not regulate massage therapists as health care practitioners, simply ask your clients whether or not they believe that massage assists them in maintaining their goals for health. Research suggests that nearly all will say yes. In a consumer survey conducted in August 2003, 90% of the respondents agreed that massage can be beneficial to one's health; 97% of 18- to 34-year-olds agreed with this statement.[1]

Unequivocally, massage makes our bodies feel better and improves our outlook on life. As a result, we may need to adopt the standards of the health care profession until the laws catch up with our professional values.

In keeping with health care standards, massage therapists must record information about their clients' health and the services provided. Obviously, treatment for healthy or injury-free clients may not require extensive documentation on a SOAP note, as does charting client symptoms and pathophysiological findings. Documenting massage therapy sessions for healthy clients is brief in comparison, and the format can be tailored to specific environments, such as spas, airport concession areas, and sporting events.

WISE ONE SPEAKS
Cost Benefits of Wellness Programs

A study described in *Wellness Management*, a newsletter of the National Wellness Association, reported the following benefits at more than 30 companies that had studied the effects of wellness programs over a 15-year period:
- **Average days of sick leave reduced by 22%**
- **Number of hospital admissions reduced by 62%**
- **Number of physician visits reduced by 16%**
- **Per capita health costs reduced by 28%**
- **Injury incidence reduced by 25%**
- **Per capita workers compensation cost reduced by 47%**

Reprinted with permission from Working in a wellness setting: New opportunities to expand your practice. Washington Massage Journal November/December 2003.

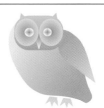

Wellness Format for Documenting Healthy Clients

A simple system for documenting healthy client sessions is **Wellness charting**. A Wellness chart contains a brief intake questionnaire for gathering health history information (Hx) and provides space for recording the treatment provided (Tx). Additional information—such as personal preferences, variations from the routine, or client progress—can be recorded in the comments section (C). The figures are optional and are useful for charting the therapist's findings, such as muscle tension and postural deviations, for clients receiving ongoing care. Three styles of Wellness charts are described in this book: (1) Standard charts for relaxation, spa therapies, and energy work; (2) Seated charts for on-site sessions; and

Wellness charting: recording of client history, all treatment provided, and additional comments regarding client preferences, practitioner findings, self-care education, and the like; also used to document wellness sessions with healthy clients

(3) Sports charts for sporting events. (Blank forms are located in the Appendix: Blank Forms on p. 10)

There are only two requirements for charting wellness sessions. First, an adequate health history is needed to ensure the client's safety (see Chapter 3). Second, it is necessary to have a detailed record of the therapy. Wellness charts must provide a historical record of wellness and health challenges over time and recount the role of the massage therapist in the client's progress toward health. The three components of treatment are:

◆ Type of massage—techniques and modalities used
◆ Location—area of massage application
◆ Duration—length of session

Treatment options in the Wellness chart can be designed so that the practitioner simply checks off or circles answers. Narrative charting is too time-consuming for fast-paced environments with high turnover. One way to speed up charting is to provide yourself with pre-determined options for treatment routines. For example, pre-event or post-event might be the only categories for a sporting event; stress buster, smooth and soothe, or energizer for an airport concession area; or seaweed wrap, mud pack, or herbal moisturizer for a salon. Time can be noted in 15-minute increments. Location can be simplified with a checklist for

full body (FB)

upper extremities (UE)

lower extremities (LE)

upper trunk (UT)

lower trunk (LT)

Customize your chart to fit your practice (see Figure 4-1).

As covered in Chapter 3, health information forms are completed annually. Modify the Wellness chart for repeat clients by eliminating the health history section and multiplying the section that records the treatment and comments. Four massage sessions can be recorded on each page (see Figure 4-2). Make a point of recording pertinent client data on the figures for

---

FIGURE 4–1 Customized Form—Sample

3. Are you allergic to any of the following? (Please circle all that apply.) Almond Oil, Aloe Vera, Cucumber, Honey, Lavender, Milk, Mud, Olive Oil, Sandalwood, Seaweed.

4. I have provided all my known medical information. I give my consent to receive treatment.
   Signature _____ Date _____

Tx: ☐ body scrub ☐ herbal wrap ☐ Swedish massage ☐ mud pack

☐ FB ☐ UE ☐ LE ☐ UT ☐ LT ☐ facial ☐ foot reflexology

C: _____

☐ 15 ☐ 30 ☐ 45 ☐ 60 minute session   initials _____ date _____

FIGURE 4–2 Seated Wellness Chart—Page 2

Massage Therapist _____   **WELLNESS CHART—SEATED**

Name _____ ID#/DOB _____ Meds _____

Tx: _____   Tx: _____

C: _____   C: _____

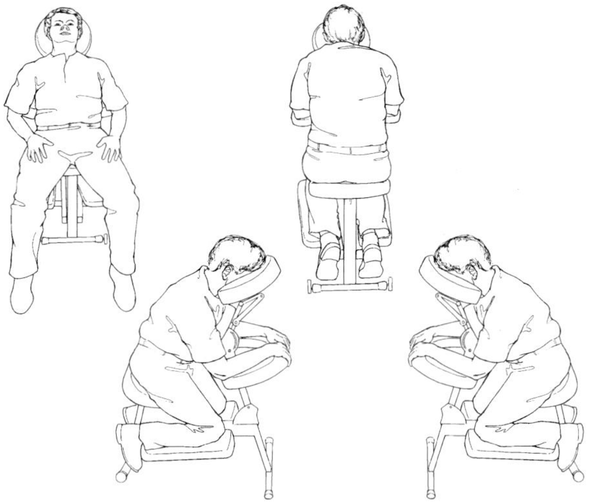

date _____ initials _____   date _____ initials _____

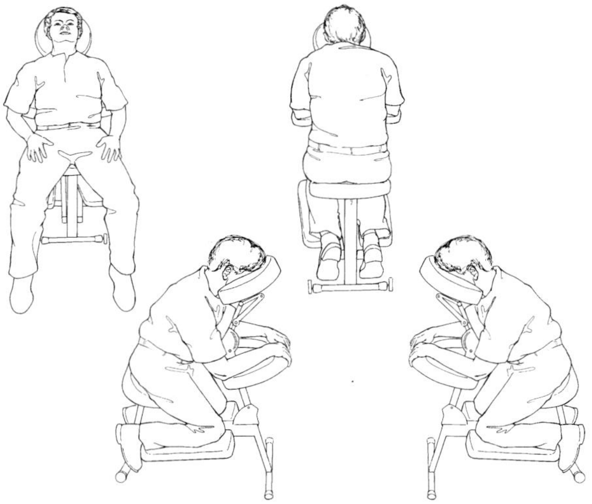

Tx: _____   Tx: _____

C: _____   C: _____

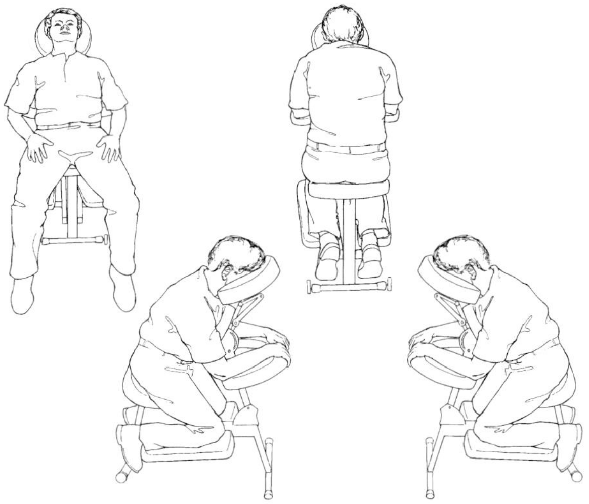

date _____ initials _____   date _____ initials _____

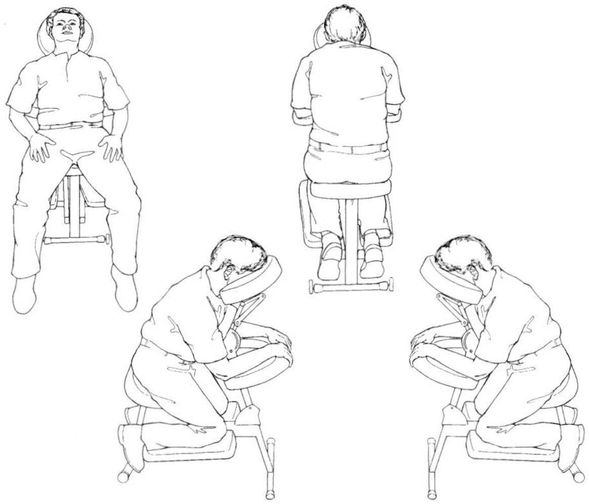

Legend:

℮ TP	● TeP	○ Ⓟ	✳ Infl	≡ HT	≈ SP
✕ Adh	≋ Numb	↻ rot	∕ elev	⊱ Short	⟷ Long

61

repeat clients. It is a quick and easy way to create a complete and accurate picture of your clients' health over time. This is useful for ongoing massage therapy sessions. It highlights problem areas and can demonstrate steady progress or recurring problems at a glance.

SOAP Charting versus Wellness Charting

With each new client, determine whether a SOAP note is necessary or whether a Wellness chart can be used. The question is not whether to document, but rather which documentation format to use—SOAP, Wellness, narrative, or others. It is always necessary to chart massage therapy sessions. Here are factors to consider when selecting one style of documentation over another:

◆ Client health
◆ Client expectations
◆ Goals of treatment
◆ Treatment results
◆ Reimbursement for services

GUIDELINES FOR SELECTING SOAP FORMAT

SOAP charting is your best option any time extensive documentation is necessary. If any one of the following statements apply, use the standard SOAP format to document the treatment. (See Chapter 5 for in-depth information on SOAP charting.)

◆ The client has health problems or symptoms and is seeking treatment to relieve them.
◆ A doctor referred the client for treatment.
◆ Insurance is involved in reimbursement.
◆ The treatment provided varies from individual to individual and is based upon client symptoms, conditions, and practitioner findings.
◆ The treatment results are significant, specific, and measurable.

A SOAP note is appropriate when the client has health concerns that the massage therapist is expected to address during treatment. SOAP charts record client symptoms and functional limitations and objective data such as inflammation, muscle spams, and trigger points. If the client is healthy, there will be no symptoms to record, no data to collect, and no condition to treat. However, clients have expectations that are sometimes similar and sometimes different than ours regarding treatment. We may believe we are providing massage for relaxation, but the client may have selected the treatment specifically to heal a whiplash injury, as was the case for Jose. Remember to clarify client goals and place them above our own and or educate clients on the limitations of the treatment. The key is to reach a mutual agreement regarding goals for health.

Always use a SOAP chart with a client who has been referred by an HCP. Referring providers generally have a particular outcome in mind, making a thorough assessment warranted. You can always switch to a Wellness chart once the client reaches his or her goals for health or when you discover that the client's health concerns are minimal and massage is primarily indicated for stress reduction.

When clients are seeking insurance reimbursement, support them by gathering information that will assist them in receiving payment for your services. Insurance plans typically require treatment to be medically necessary. A SOAP note will provide the documentation required to prove **medical necessity**. If you cannot find supportive data—proof of a

medical necessity: covered services required to preserve and maintain the health status of a member or eligible person in accordance with the area's standards of medical practice

medical condition that massage can treat effectively and efficiently—chart the massage sessions on a Wellness chart rather than stretching the truth simply to fill a SOAP chart.

A common mistake when using a SOAP chart to record Wellness massage is to note tight muscles as moderately or severely hypertonic, even though the client's activity level is not affected by the tight muscle. It would be more realistic to describe the tight muscles as mildly hypertonic—the tight muscle does not interfere with the client's ability to perform daily activities. Claire, in the opening story, was hoping for documentation affirming that her regular massage therapy was addressing minor tight muscles and stiff joints, not the injury treatment the insurance company inferred.

All massage therapy treatments should be modified to meet the needs of the client. The difference between a treatment that warrants a SOAP chart and one appropriate for a Wellness chart lies in the overall intent. Sessions in which treatments vary constantly based on individual symptoms and findings and are applied in a curative manner deserve a SOAP chart. For example, if cross-fiber friction is applied directly over scar tissue with the intent to decrease adhesions and increase mobility, the treatment has curative intent and should be recorded on a SOAP chart. Massage routines that vary slightly and occur in every session—as when modifications are made to ensure client safety and comfort, such as adjusting positions or providing a pillow—do not require a SOAP chart.

Treatment results that go beyond general therapeutic benefits, such as decreasing pain, increasing postural balance, or increasing mobility, should be substantiated on a SOAP chart. Document progress by measuring significant changes in subjective and objective findings. If, for example, you and your client initially determined that treatment was strictly for general health purposes—increasing muscle relaxation, circulation, and energy—and you have been using the Wellness charting method, switch to the SOAP format once you and the client determine that the goals of the therapy have changed.

Organize the charts in the client's file chronologically by date regardless of format. There is no need to keep SOAP notes separate from Wellness notes. It is acceptable to mix charting formats within a single file. Clients often fluxuate between wellness care and treatment massage as their needs change and they reach their goals for health.

GUIDELINES FOR SELECTING WELLNESS FORMAT

Use Wellness charting when the client is healthy, when treatment is routine, and when sessions are not used as ongoing, curative health care. Follow these guidelines for determining whether a session warrants this style of documentation:

◆ The client is healthy and has no specific health issues.
◆ If the client has health issues, the specific health conditions, symptoms, and findings are not addressed in the session other than for client safety and comfort.
◆ Treatment is provided for general therapeutic benefits—such as improved circulation, relaxation, and energy—without the intent or expectation of altering existing health conditions or symptoms such as localized pain, numbness, compensatory postural patterns, or limited mobility.
◆ The treatment is routine. The practitioner does not deviate from that routine except to ensure client safety and comfort, regardless of symptoms and pathophysiological findings.
◆ The client is not using the session as ongoing, curative health care treatment for a specific condition.

RELAXATION THERAPIES: SOAP OR WELLNESS?

The style and the intent of the treatment can determine the documentation format. Drainage techniques applied as a full-body routine with general circulatory benefits may warrant Wellness charting. A drainage session designed to treat inflammation resulting from a swollen ankle warrants SOAP charting. Massage modalities, such as Trager, Swedish massage, and Polarity can be applied with either curative or palliative intent. Follow the guidelines outlined earlier to determine whether to use SOAP charting or Wellness charting. Use the Standard Wellness chart for documenting most relaxation therapies (see Figure 4-3).

In many cases, the guidelines for determining an appropriate charting format are easy to apply. However, situations exist in which the lines blur. For example, many massage therapists find it impossible to follow a relaxation routine and not address what they feel underneath their hands. If you find yourself treating specific findings and straying from a routine, note the variations from the routine and the objective findings in the comments section of the Wellness chart. If the client returns for additional treatment, and together you make the decision toward a more detailed treatment plan, switch to a SOAP format.

Relaxation is a general health benefit with widespread effects. Simple effleurage strokes can have profound analgesic results. Basic gymnastics can produce dramatic changes in mobility and function. Symptoms have been shown to resolve and illnesses to go into remission from healing touch.[2] The intent in providing an abbreviated format for charting is not to belittle the magnitude of hands-on healing, but rather to provide an avenue to simplify the paperwork when appropriate. Use the Wellness format when the treatment is intended to be palliative, not curative. If the results are more profound than anticipated, describe them in the comments section.

ENERGY WORK: SOAP OR WELLNESS?

Energy work, like any other massage therapy, can be charted on either a SOAP note or an Wellness chart, depending on the condition of the client and the intent of the treatment. The challenge in using a SOAP format to record energy work is one of language rather than style. Objective findings are not as tangible to the untrained hand or eye, but they are equally valid. The initial challenge is to come up with a vocabulary to define what you feel and see and to use it consistently and in a way that makes sense to others who are untrained in energetic modalities. The list of abbreviations provided at the end of this book contains standard symbols and abbreviations for energetic findings and treatment techniques (see Appendix: Abbreviations List). Create an addendum for additional terms to fit your practice or list additional terms directly on the Wellness chart (see Figure 4-4).

Guidelines for documenting energy work: Follow the guidelines for selecting the style of documentation. If Wellness charting is appropriate, chart the treatment routine and note the client's response to treatment in the comments section or near the data noted on the human figures (see Figure 4-4). If SOAP charting is necessary, follow the guidelines presented in the next chapter. Here is a modified summary of what you will find in Chapter 5, regarding the charting of energy work:

◆ S—Note subjective information as defined in Chapter 5.
◆ O—Note objective findings specific to your energetic training. Emphasize physiological findings. Use common terminology whenever possible.
◆ O—State treatment location, duration, and modalities used. Highlight specifics.

FIGURE 4–3 Standard Wellness Chart—Relaxation

Naomi Wachtel
567 Sunnydale Dr.
Flat Irons, CO   80302
TEL   303 555 8866

WELLNESS CHART

Name _Lin Pak_____ ID#/DOB _5-31-63_____ Date _7-27-04____

Phone _(303) 555-0033x253_____ Address _IBM 3rd Floor_____

1. What are your goals for health, and how may I assist you in achieving your goals? _Limit___
long-term complications of diabetes through relaxation and stress reduction

2. List typical daily activities—work, exercise, home. _I sit a lot at work and watch movies___
_____at home_

3. Are you currently experiencing any of the following? If yes, please explain.

   pain, tenderness   ☒ No ☐ Yes: _____   stiffness ☒ No ☐ Yes: _____
   numbness or tingling ☒ No ☐ Yes: _____   swelling ☒ No ☐ Yes: _____
   allergies   ☒ No ☐ Yes: _____

4. List all illnesses, injuries, and health concerns you have now or have had in the past 3 years.
   (Examples: arthritis, diabetes, car crash, pregnancy) _diabetes, borderline high blood___
   pressure

5. List medications and pain relievers taken this week. _insulin_____

6. I have provided all my known medical information. I acknowledge that massage therapy is
   not a substitute for medical diagnosis and treatment. I give my consent to receive treatment.

   Signature _Lin Pak_____ Date _7-27-04____

   Tx: _Full Body Swedish Massage, Lymph Drainage trunk and upper extremities_____
   _____45-minute session_

   C: _Homework-relaxation exercises, check blood pressure before and after_____
   _____massages at home_

Legend:

℮ TP	● TeP	○ ℗	✳ Infl	≡ HT	≈ SP	initials _NW, LMT_
✕ Adh	≋ Numb	⟲ rot	╱ elev	⊢⊣ Short	⟷ Long	

65

FIGURE 4-4 Standard Wellness Chart—Energy Work

Naomi Wachtel
567 Sunnydale Dr.
Flat Irons, CO   80302
Tᴇʟ   303 555 8866

WELLNESS CHART

Name _Lin Pak_   ID#/DOB _5-31-63_   Meds _insulin_

Tx: _60 minute Polarity and Somato-_   Tx: _____
      Emotional Release, FB

C: _↑ balance 3rd chakra, shoulder posture,_   C: _____
      ↓ fascial pull

_Y_ fascial
   shortening

      congestion

        ↘ rotation

date _08-03-04_   initials _NW, LMT_   date _____   initials _____

- O—State measurable changes in the subjective and objective data as a result of the session. Gauge the changes in intensity and quality of expression. Describe how the changes affect the client's quality of life?
- A—If the client's ability to function in everyday activities is impaired, set goals based on improving function, as defined in Chapter 5.
- P—Create a treatment plan and provide self-care instructions, as described in Chapter 5.

Energy work is controversial among insurance companies as a reimbursable treatment modality because treatment results have not been adequately substantiated scientifically. This is also the case with other massage modalities. Lymphatic drainage is one of the few massage modalities to date with substantial international scientific evidence of effectiveness.[3] As a result, demonstrating measurable progress based in function, symptoms, and physiological findings is important for all massage modalities. When charting energy work or emotional bodywork, emphasize the physical expressions of the energetic or emotional dysfunction. Emphasize the results of treatment over the modalities used. Use terminology that is easily understood across professions.

Venues Befitting Wellness Charting

There are many venues in which Wellness charting is appropriate. Two common ones are sporting events, in which participants receive pre-event or post-event therapy, and spas, in which clients self-select from a menu of treatments designed for relaxation, detoxification, and beautification. The purpose of these sessions is specific to the venue, not to the individual, and the treatment routines do not vary much. Because these routines address general therapeutic goals and are not tailored to individual needs, clients are not likely to depend on them for ongoing health care.

Each venue has specific documentation needs. The following will be addressed individually:

◆ Events—such as sporting events, and health fairs
◆ On-site venues—such as offices, malls, airports, and grocery stores
◆ Spas and salons

EVENT THERAPY

A common sight near the finish line at foot races or under a tent at street fairs is a large group of massage therapists with tables or chairs providing relief for participants. Massage therapy offered at venues like these—sporting events, health fairs, and community events—require Wellness charting. The pace is fast, the turnover is frequent, the sessions are brief, and the need to document is minimal. The charts will not become permanent records of the clients' health, nor will the information be used for ongoing care. But the charts do assist the practitioner in determining whether treatment is appropriate, and they provide a record that will become crucial if the client claims to have been injured in the course of treatment.

Treatment provided at events meets the guidelines for alternative charting. The clients are healthy enough to be competing physically. Therapists are there to provide basic services and a routine treatment. People are generally not seeking curative health care at these venues, and practitioners do not have the time or information necessary to treat specific health conditions. Although therapists may use the event as an opportunity to market their practices, for many it is the only treatment the client will receive from this therapist. If the client does seek out the therapist's professional services in the future, a formal intake will ensue and a decision will be made at that time whether SOAP notes or Wellness notes will be appropriate for ongoing care.

Because the pace is fast and distractions are many at an event, you should read the intake questions aloud to the client. Make eye contact to ensure that the client is paying attention and is understanding the questions being asked. If the client answers yes to any of the questions, the practitioner must be prepared to ask additional questions that are not on the intake form to establish the appropriateness of treatment. For example, if the client says he has swollen feet, rule out infections and heart conditions that could be exacerbated by treatment. If the client was injured recently, determine whether alternative treatment methods are appropriate and whether treatment to certain areas of the body should be avoided.[4] If the client has just finished a race and is exhibiting signs of shock, first aid should be administered immediately in the medical tent. As discussed in Chapter 3, the intake information is brief but critical in event venues. Tailor your event Wellness chart to the specific venue and the treatment routines you provide.

The nature of massage therapy at events is that there are no repeat visits. The event occurs once, or annually, and the tables and chairs are packed up and gone by the next day. As a result, several client sessions can be recorded on one form—individual client files need not be created. The intake questions top the form and are read to each individual, and space is provided below to record the athlete's name, the positive responses to intake questions, and the treatment provided, including modalities, location, and duration.

ON-SITE MASSAGE

On-site massage is increasingly popular in work environments as an employee benefit. Many businesses recognize the detrimental effects of stress on job performance and long-term health[5] and offer on-site massage in an effort to keep productivity high and reduce sick leave.

On-site massage differs from event massage in one important way—the site is often permanent. On-site companies or individual practitioners contract with businesses for regular visits, often weekly. When massage is a regular fixture in the work environment—accessible, non-threatening, and affordable—clients who might not otherwise seek the services of a massage therapist may become repeat customers. A permanent site with repeat customers, many of whom have symptoms of repetitive stress conditions, presents some charting challenges, given the time constraints of on-site massage environments.

On-site massage, similar to event therapy, is fast-paced, has high turnover, and involves brief treatments. There is no time for extensive interviews, intake forms, or breaks between sessions for charting. However, the need for documentation is great. Charting must be quick and easy, and it must serve the needs of the client.

In an interview, David Palmer, often called the father of on-site massage, said, "I don't see on-site massage . . . too closely associated with health care services because it's not a treatment . . . It's not designed to fix anything. It's merely designed to make people feel better and to produce what I think is the greatest value of massage, which is to simply enhance circulation."[6] In such situations, a brief Wellness chart is adequate. However, some people in the workplace have carpal tunnel syndrome, chronic headaches, or fibromyalgia. Many of those people use the on-site massage provided in their offices to treat their symptoms and keep them functioning productively in the workplace. A record of their symptoms, physiological findings, and progress could benefit both the practitioner and the clients. Demonstrating tangible results to the business owners and to the clients will increase customer satisfaction, demand, and availability.

The Seated Wellness chart provides an alternative to the Sports Wellness chart (see Figure 4-5). The primary addition to the chart are illustrations of a person in a treatment chair. The practitioner draws symbols on the human figures and quickly charts symptoms and objective findings, creating an easy reference for demonstrating progress and planning future treatments. The Seated Wellness chart contains an intake form, records measurable subjective and objective data, notes treatment routines, and provides space for additional comments from the practitioner.

FIGURE 4-5 Seated Wellness Chart—Page I

Sarah Benjamin
123 Sun Moon and Stars Drive
Capital Hill, WA   98119
Tel   206 555 4446

WELLNESS CHART—SEATED

Name __Tham Maad__   ID#/DOB __12-19-80__   Date __12-12-04__

Phone __ext 134__   Address __Microtech N. campus 2nd floor__

1. What are your goals for health, and how may I assist you in achieving your goals? _____
   __work without numbness, relax__

2. List typical daily activities—work, exercise, home. __computer, reading, skateboarding__

3. Are you currently experiencing any of the following? If yes, please explain.

pain, tenderness	☒ No ☐ Yes: _____	stiffness ☐ No ☒ Yes: __R SH__
numbness or tingling	☐ No ☒ Yes: __R hand__	swelling ☒ No ☐ Yes: _____
allergies	☒ No ☐ Yes: _____	

4. List all illnesses, injuries, and health concerns you have now or have had in the past 3 years.
   (Examples: arthritis, diabetes, car crash, pregnancy) __MVC Aug. 1993__

5. List medications and pain relievers taken this week. __none__

6. I have provided all my known medical information. I acknowledge that massage therapy is
   not a substitute for medical diagnosis and treatment. I give my consent to receive treatment.

   Signature __Tham Maad__   Date __12-12-04__

   Tx: __30 min. SW (M) - Focus on (R) SH, arm, hand, BL neck, chest, back, light pressure__

   C: __tingling in (R) hand radiates from (R) elbow, intermittant, worse in AM and late afternoon__

MΔL
  X

L
Δ
N

MΔL
  X
  X
≋L⁺ΔL

MΔL⁺

initials __SB, UMT__

Legend:
ℰ TP   ● TeP   ○ Ⓟ   ⋇ Infl   ≡ HT   ≈ SP
✕ Adh   ≋ Numb   ↻ rot   ╱ elev   ⤜ Short   ↔ Long

Several treatments for the same client may be recorded on Page 2 of the Seated Wellness chart, preventing repetitive health-information gathering (refer to Figure 4-2). As with events, on-site venues such as airports, convention centers, shopping malls, and grocery stores are not prone to repeat clientele. The clientele is transient, the desire to receive treatment is spontaneous, and sessions are routine. Do not attempt to record repeat visits for on-site clients. File charts by date, rather than by client name, and have each client fill out a new intake with each visit. Use Page 1 of the Seated Wellness chart for these venues (Figure 4-5) or custom design a Wellness chart that meets your individual needs.

SPA AND SALON SESSIONS

Spas are traditionally located in resorts that cater to a transient population. More and more, however, spas are found in downtown areas, urban neighborhoods, and inside salons. Salons are incorporating massage and hydrotherapy with traditional pedicures, manicures, and facials. With increasing availability, people are becoming regular beneficiaries of massage therapies in spas.

Spas and salons are ideal environments for Wellness charting. The need for extensive charting is low, and the turnover is fast. Treatment is routine and consistent, varying little with individual needs. Clients select treatment routines from a menu, based on the general health benefits advertised. The primary role for massage therapy in a spa environment is for pampering, relaxing, cleansing, detoxifying, and toning the skin. Clients rarely consider the treatment to be a remedy for illnesses or injuries.

The use of the Wellness chart in spas and salons is simple and practical. Practitioners use the chart to identify health conditions that contraindicate extreme temperatures or increases in circulation. Skin allergies and sensitivities are also major concerns when gathering health history. Treatment options are checked off, and comments primarily reflect the personal preferences of the clients. Use the Standard Wellness chart (see Figure 4-3) or design a Spa Wellness chart to meet your individual needs.

Space is provided on a single chart for multiple sessions, because clients may return. In a curative health care environment, client visits are weekly or biweekly. In a spa environment, monthly or quarterly visits are the norm.

SUMMARY

Document all massage therapy sessions. Two options for charting are:

◆ SOAP charting
◆ Wellness charting

Use the Wellness format for relaxation treatments and energy work—depending on the health of the client and the intent of the treatment—and in the following venues:

◆ Events, such as sporting events and health fairs
◆ On-site locations, such as offices, malls, and airports
◆ Spas and salons

To ensure the effectiveness of the Wellness chart, vary the intake questions and treatment options according to the venue and the practitioner's treatment style. Use the Wellness format for charting sessions that meet the following guidelines:

◆ The client is healthy and has no specific health issues.
◆ If the client has health issues, the specific health conditions, symptoms, and findings are not addressed in the session.
◆ Treatment is provided for general therapeutic benefits without the intent or expectation of altering health problems or symptoms.
◆ The treatment is routine.
◆ The client is not using the session as ongoing, curative health care treatment for a specific condition.

REFERENCES

1. Opinion Research Corporation International. Hands On: The Newsletter of the American Massage Therapy Association, November/December 2003.
2. Carson R, Shield B. Healers on Healing. Los Angeles, CA: Tarcher Inc., 1989.
3. Chikly B. Silent Waves: Theory and Practice of Lymphatic Drainage Therapy. Scottsdale, AZ: I.H.H. Publishing, 2002.
4. Werner R. A Massage Therapist's Guide to Pathology, 2nd Ed. Baltimore, MD: Williams & Wilkins, 2002.
5. Hafen BQ, Karren KJ, Frandsen KJ, Smith NL. Mind Body Health: The Effects of Attitudes, Emotions, and Relationships. Boston: Allyn & Bacon, 1996.
6. Mower M. The on-site massage movement: Interviews with David Palmer, Russ Borner, Raymond Blaylock. Massage Magazine March/April 1994.

Documentation: SOAP Charting

CHAPTER OUTLINE

A medical director of an insurance carrier in Idaho was questioned by a group of massage therapists: "Why isn't massage therapy a covered benefit in any of your plans?" He replied, "If every massage therapist can show me six months of SOAP charts on every client, we will consider it."

Introduction

SOAP (Subjective, Objective, Assessment, Plan) charting is a standard format for documenting treatment sessions in the health care field. It is routinely used by physicians, physical therapists, chiropractors, nurses, massage therapists, and other medical and allied health professionals.[1] The rapid and widespread adoption of the SOAP format is a tribute to its simple structure and inherent flexibility. Any health concern, method of evaluation, and treatment style can be recorded in the SOAP format. The SOAP structure meets the needs of a variety of health care professionals in many settings.

The SOAP chart documents the client's health information and goals, the practitioner's findings and treatment, and the client's self-care routine; and records the client's response to the solutions and progress toward the goals. The information is organized into four categories:

- **S**ubjective—data provided by the client (symptoms and functional limitations)
- **O**bjective—data from the practitioner's perspective (movement tests, palpation findings, visual observations, and treatment and the client's immediate response to the treatment)
- **A**ssessment—functional goals and outcomes based in activities of daily living
- **P**lan—treatment recommendations and self-care education

This structure prompts comprehensive information gathering and makes data storage and retrieval easy.

Adaptations of the SOAP format have been created for massage therapists, for example SOTxAP[2] and CARE.[3] This chapter provides basic information for massage therapists on how to use the traditional SOAP format with a focus on **functional outcomes reporting**. Some clinics, hospitals, and schools may require a standard of documentation that varies slightly from that presented here; however, the skills acquired through this text can be easily adapted to suit any system of documentation. When message therapists master the basics most common to all health care providers, the transition will be easy when an employer requires another format or the therapist chooses something more appropriate for his or her needs. For example, SOAP charting can be adapted into the CARE format, as noted below:

- **C**ondition of the client—measurable data regarding the client's medical condition, such as pain or tension (traditionally split between the Subjective and Objective sections)
- **A**ction taken—types of massage provided, location, and duration of treatment (part of the Objective section)
- **R**esponse of client—measurable physiological changes, verbal and non-verbal feedback (Assessment—proponents of CARE charting do not advocate using the functional outcomes style of reporting)
- **E**valuation—recommendations for future treatment, such as massage, client homework, and suggestions to other caregivers (Plan)

functional outcomes reporting: style of charting that addresses (1) client's ability to function in everyday activities, (2) goal setting, and (3) treatment design to improve function and motivate increased client participation

74

The advantages of using the SOAP format include:

◆ Consistency across professions
◆ Common language and communication style
◆ Demonstration of professionalism
◆ Proof of progress and functional outcomes
◆ Brevity and comprehensiveness
◆ Fast retrieval of information

Another recent trend in documentation is functional outcomes reporting. This style of charting—writing notes that address the client's ability to function in everyday activities and setting goals and designing treatments to improve function—is quickly being adopted by physical therapists and massage therapists. Functional outcomes reporting fits into the SOAP format and shifts the focus of documentation to the client's quality of life. The practitioner records the client's functional limitations and works with the client to develop goals for returning to personally meaningful activities, and together, the practitioner and client implement solutions to reach those goals. Because this style of recording information is client-focused, relying less on the diagnostic capabilities of the practitioner, it is a natural addition to the charting regimen for massage therapists and is therefore emphasized in this book.

Guidelines for Charting

First and foremost, charting should contribute to the therapeutic relationship, not detract from it. Don't let charting be a distraction. Follow the client's lead in the interview.[4] You do not need to follow the SOAP format in order. The beauty of the SOAP structure is that you can organize your information in a linear fashion without having to think or speak in a linear manner. As information is presented, place it in the appropriate section.

Be attentive and maintain good listening skills, as discussed in Chapter 1. If the client is emotional and needs your undivided attention, record the information later. It is more important to be attentive to the client in a moment of need than to write on the chart. Reflect your understanding of the client's experience after she is composed and record the data appropriate to her health concerns once she verifies the information.

Be brief. Jot down just enough to jog your memory later, such as words, dates, or short phrases.[5] It can be difficult to discern important information about the client's health as you are listening to her story. Things often make more sense later, after you have heard the whole story. Take brief notes and fill in the blanks after you summarize the pertinent information to the client and get confirmation of your interpretation. Make sure you accurately represent the client's concerns.

Measure everything. Gather as much detail as possible to document the injury or health concern—and write it down. It is difficult to prove progress when there is nothing to mark progress against. For example, pain may still be present but diminished, occurring less frequently, with a shorter duration and fewer exacerbations than at the previous session. Be thorough. If information is worth writing down, it is worth measuring.

Avoid vague statements. It is not enough to write "feeling better," "condition is improved," or "pain increases with sitting." Be specific. Rate the intensity of pain, describe the activities that are limited, and state how long the client is able do the activity before the symptoms increase or the activity must cease. Use measurable data to explain the symptoms and compare the symptoms to those from the previous session to demonstrate progress. For example: Mild pain, intermittant, increasing to moderate pain with sitting for one hour or more expresses a decrease in pain when compared with last week's SOAP note: Moderate pain, constant, unable to sit for 30 minutes or more. The information should be able to stand alone. "Feeling better" is not only vague, but it can be taken out of context and can signal to an insurance company to discontinue care because she no longer requires treatment.[6]

Use consistent terminology to measure your findings and client symptoms, such as mild, moderate, or severe. It is difficult to note progress when comparing "hurts pretty bad" to "kinda sore or sorta achy." If you are unclear about the best term to use that fits the patient's symptoms, use these guidelines:

◆ Mild, or 1, 2, or 3 out of 10 describes the severity of a symptom, but that the symptom does not interfere with the patient's ability to function. Zero out of 10 is synonymous with normal or within normal limits.

◆ Moderate, or 4, 5, or 6 out of 10 describes the severity of a symptom, and as a result of that symptom, the patient is forced to modify daily activities.

◆ Severe, or 7, 8, or 9 out of 10 describes the severity of a symptom, and as a result of that symptom, the patient is unable to perform some activities of daily living. Ten out of 10 is reserved for clients who are bedridden or disabled as a result of that symptom.

Chart only information applicable to the client's condition and goals for health. Often, a story surrounds pertinent details. Pay attention to the details of the story, but be selective when choosing the information to document. Record only data that substantiate the concern or contribute to the solution. For example, Lin experiences an increase in allergies at work when Sally, a coworker from marketing, wears heavy perfume. It is not important to mention information about work or the coworker. The important thing to note is that Lin's allergy symptoms increase when exposed to perfume.

Be objective. State everything in a factual manner. Leave your opinions off the chart. For example, omit "I think the client doesn't want to get better and is avoiding going back to work." Instead, quote the client directly in the Subjective section. He may comment on the situation in ways that adequately represent his state of mind, opinions, or emotions. Chart specific, measurable information and let his lack of progress, as an example, demonstrate that the treatment is not producing results. The information should pertain to the client, not to you.[6] Revisit the discussion in Chapter 1: If the relationship isn't productive, step up the communication and reconsider your approach.

As you ask the client specific questions—to confirm an assessment or rule out a particular condition—record the positive and negative findings. Negative findings include, for example: All active cervical ranges of motion (ROM) normal . . . The positive finding: . . . except left lateral flexion—moderately limited with mild pain at tissue stretch. If the negative findings are not recorded, it will be difficult to remember 30 days later, at the reevaluation session, which ROM tests were done at the initial assessment.

Consider another example in which "no" answers are as important as "yes" answers: Jose has shoulder pain. The pain increases when he raises his arm to the side, but there is no pain with any other shoulder movement. Knowing that there is no pain with a particular action—if you are identifying a rotator cuff injury or determining bursitis versus tendonitis—could affect your treatment plan as much as knowing that there is pain with an action. Record all answers that contribute to the case. Even if your scope of practice does not permit you to state on your SOAP note whether the client has bursitis or tendonitis, the information is critical to your treatment plan: Bursitis and tendonitis are treated very differently. State only that there is pain with all ranges of motion, not that the client has bursitis, unless you have diagnostic scope and can treat accordingly.

Use common medical terms and become fluent with standard abbreviations (see Appendix: Abbreviations List). Many standardized medical abbreviations and symbols used by all types of health care providers (HCP) are applicable to massage therapy. The medical terms referred to here are descriptive, not diagnostic. Use terms familiar to the health care community to describe your findings, such as hypertonic (HT), spastic (SP), fibrotic (fib), ischemic (IS); rather than tight, lumpy, ropey, or mushy. Use the shorthand available for these terms to make charting quick and easy.

▼

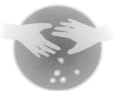

BONE GAME
Translation

Headache pain, pounding, left frontal, moderate minus, 2 to 3 days, monthly, with menses for 10 plus years.

Abbreviation: HA Ⓟ, pounding, Ⓛ frontal, M–, 2–3 day/mth, c̄ menses 10+ yr

The trigger point was moderately painful with digital pressure at the trigger point site and mildly painful at the referral site.

Abbreviation: TP M Ⓟ c̄ dig. pres. @ TP site & L Ⓟ @ ref. site

Cervical flexion passive range of motion was limited moderate minus with mild pain at end range.

Abbreviation: C-flex P-ROM↓M– c̄ L Ⓟ @ end range

Right shoulder active abduction moderate segmented movement with mild compensational shoulder elevation at end range.

Abbreviation: Ⓡsh-abd A-ROMM seg c̄ L comp. sh-elev @ end range.

Moderate trigger point site pain changed to mild pain, mild referred pain changed to no pain.

Abbreviation: TP site M Ⓟ Δ L Ⓟ, L ref. Ⓟ Δ Ⓟ̸

Moderate segmented movement in right shoulder active abduction changed to smooth movement without compensational shoulder elevation.

Abbreviation: M seg. mvm't Ⓡsh-abd A-ROM Δsm s̄ comp. sh-elev

Client supine, anterior-lateral view, deep inhalation, mild plus mobility restriction upper right.

Abbreviation: pt supine, ant-lat view, deep inhal., ↓ mob L+ upper Ⓡ

Left biceps insertion moderate pain with mild digital pressure, mild plus referred pain into left elbow.

Abbreviation: Ⓛ biceps insert. M Ⓟ c̄ L dig. pres., L+ ref. Ⓟ → Ⓛ elbow

1-hour full-body Swedish massage; 30-minute foot reflexology; or 90-minute Hellerwork—inspiration.

Abbreviation: 1 hr FB Sw Ⓜ; 30 min foot reflex.; 90 min HW—inspir.

Muscle energy with cervical flexion, direct pressure on scalene trigger point, or myofascial release on diaphragm.

Abbreviation: MET c̄ C-flex, DP scal. TP, MFR diaph.

Craniosacral therapy with attention to the thoracic cage, muscle energy for cervical flexion and extension, and lymph drainage for upper trunk and head.

Abbreviation: CST T cage, MET C-flex & ext, LDT UT & hd.

Add personalized abbreviations to the list of standard ones to meet the needs of your practice. Do not use abbreviations that are not on your list, even abbreviated words that you think are common, such as quads for quadriceps muscles or hams for hamstring muscles. Others who read the client file must be able to interpret everything on the chart. Payment of your bill may depend on a claims representative understanding your notes. If you use a series of tests or treatment techniques that do not have standard abbreviations, create your own shorthand and produce a legend to attach to the standardized list. For example, many of Sari's clients have been in motor vehicle collisions (MVC). She finds it helpful to abbreviate information regarding the crash and whiplash-related injuries, but the abbreviations list she uses does not have the medical terms she requires for her practice. Therefore, she includes her own shorthand legend with the standard list she sends out when her charts are requested (see Figure 5-1).

Never use correction fluid or an eraser to eliminate information. Cross out mistakes with a single line. Initial and date the error. Do not leave blank spaces where data could be altered (see Amending the Forms section in Chapter 3).

Sign your legal name or initials at the end of every chart entry. Never use nicknames—SOAP charts are legal documents. Stay current with legal-name changes, which are common with marriage or divorce. Include your health care credentials with your signature. The supervising practitioner signs the chart in addition to student, aide, or apprentice in learning environments or clinic settings.[6]

Write legibly. Insurance carriers can refuse payment if they are unable to ascertain whether the treatment was reasonable and necessary, or whether the symptoms warranted the type of treatment.[6] Chart notes are the primary source for verifying this information. If the notes are illegible, payment can legitimately be denied. Charting is intended to facilitate

FIGURE 5–1 Motor Vehicle Collision Treatment and Billing Abbreviations	
accel	acceleration
CADS	cervical acceleration deceleration syndrome
CPT	Current Procedural Terminology
G-Force	acceleration force
HCFA-1500	Health Care Financing Administration current billing form
HCP	health care provider
ICD	International Classification for Disease
IME	independent medical examination
MVC	motor vehicle collision
PCP	primary care provider
PIP	personal injury protection
PR	peer review
pre-IS	pre-injury status
pre-XC	pre-existing conditions
+SB	wearing seat belt
SB-	not wearing seat belt
WAS	whiplash associated disorder

communication. Make it easy for others to read the information you are trying to share. It is acceptable for your signature to be illegible. Just make sure you have your name, address, and phone number stamped clearly on each page in the client's file so others can determine who the practitioner is and how to contact you.

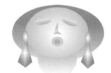

STORY TELLER
Who to Pay?

An insurance adjuster called needing more information on a client before she could authorize payment. She couldn't read the client's name written on the SOAP chart, and there was no identifying information about the client, such as insurance identification number or date of birth. I asked her to fax me the charts because I couldn't place who the client might be. As the charts came over the fax, I was taken aback. The handwriting was not mine. The initials signing the chart entries were not mine, and the client was not mine! The charts were not only missing client information, there was no contact information for the massage therapist. The only legible name on the chart was mine—next to the little copyright symbol (©) in the lower right hand corner of the form. I tried to explain to her that I created the form, but I did not write the chart note. I don't know if the correct massage therapist was ever paid for her services.

Components of SOAP Format

Subjective, Objective, Assessment, Plan (SOAP) notes were created as part of a documentation system called the **problem-oriented medical record (POMR)**, introduced by Dr. Lawrence Weed in the 1960s. Historically, the POMR listed client problems in the front of the chart, and the practitioner wrote a separate SOAP note to address each problem.[10] Currently, it is acceptable to write one SOAP note for each session, addressing all of the "problems" on the same SOAP note. The SOAP format was developed to help structure the practitioner's efforts to solve the client's health issues. The practitioner records the client's health concerns, the practitioner's findings, sets goals with the client, and develops a treatment plan based on the findings and goals. Practical and easy to use, the SOAP note has become the charting standard in the health care industry.

problem-oriented medical record (POMR): documentation system, introduced by Dr. Lawrence Weed in the 1960s, that lists the patient's problems at the front of the chart and allows a practitioner to write a SOAP note to address each problem

SUBJECTIVE

Subjective information provided by the client includes a health history and current health information. Data collected on the intake forms is considered subjective information and is used to provide comprehensive documentation of the client's health at the onset of treatment. Use the Subjective section of the SOAP chart as an ongoing record of details about the client's current health status: current concerns, physical symptoms, emotional complications, changes in functional ability, and impact on the client's daily routine.

On a SOAP chart, subjective information is divided into three parts:

◆ A prioritized list of health concerns or goals for the session
◆ Symptoms relating to the current health concerns
◆ Activities that aggravate or relieve the symptoms

Health Concerns

Place the client's health concerns at the top of the SOAP chart. Remain mindful of the reasons why the client is seeking care. The client's health concerns may be defined as injuries, medical conditions, symptoms, or as goals for maintaining health or preventing disease. For example, Darnel is seeking care for injuries sustained in a motor vehicle collision, Tham wants to be able to work without pain or numbness, and Lin is eager to prevent complications of diabetes and learn relaxation skills. Include pertinent information that directly affects the care you provide for the current date of service.

Some of the information may not come directly from the client. A prescription may provide the diagnosis, or contributing information may come from test results you did not perform. Darnel's x-rays, for example, show degenerative scoliosis; Tham has a diagnosed repetitive stress disorder; and Lin has a family history of heart disease that potentially could complicate her diabetes. This information is critical to the direction of subjective information gathering and the formation of the treatment plan, but may or may not have originated with the client. Typically, this information is found on the health information form, but if diagnoses come trickling in after the fact, write it in the Subjective section under Health Concerns. References to spinal stenosis or carpel tunnel syndrome will not be misconstrued as operating outside your scope of practice. It is appropriate to list diagnostic terms in this section of the SOAP chart, because the information comes from the client or the HCP.

Prioritize multiple concerns. For example, Darnel has limited neck range of motion, back pain, and headaches. In Chapter 1, we discussed his strong desire to reduce the back pain so he could interact with his granddaughter Madi. His headaches are more distressing than his limited neck mobility. Therefore, we would prioritize his health concerns or needs in the following order: Treat injuries and symptoms associated with the motor vehicle collision including secondary scoliosis recurrence.

1. Reduce low back pain.
2. Reduce headache pain.
3. Increase neck mobility.

It is imperative to ask clients to prioritze their health concerns, rather than to assume one symptom is more critical than another. For example, Jack has a list of four concerns he asks to be addressed in his massage: sharp pain in the right hip, low back stiffness, achy right knee, and swelling in the left thumb. Assuming that the lower body complex is the most pressing concern for Jack, his massage therapist gets busy working on the low back, hip, and knee. She does a thorough job, but runs out of time before addressing the swollen thumb. By the time Jack is up and off the table, the low back, hip, and knee feel fantastic. The massage therapist feels confident the session was a success, having accomplished three of Jack's four concerns. He, however, leaves disappointed. He knows he doesn't have a chance at winning the arm wrestling contest at the pub this weekend with a swollen thumb. Avoid any misunderstandings by asking clients to prioritize their goals for the session. In addition, review your treatment plan with them before you begin the massage.

Symptoms

Obtain a complete list of symptoms from the client in the initial interview. Much of this information is recorded on the intake forms. Synthesize and condense the information in **initial SOAP notes**. Inquire about specific areas that have bearing on your treatment

initial SOAP notes: comprehensive notes recording the patient's first visit with a practitioner for a particular condition, including exam, findings, treatment, and treatment plan regarding the patient's health and current situation

applications and are within your scope of practice. Commonly, massage therapists inquire about signs and symptoms in these categories:

- General—fatigue, pain, signs of stress, allergies, fever, posture, and general function
- Lymphatic—swollen nodes, edema
- Musculo-skeletal—tension, weakness, muscle or joint pain, stiffness, swelling
- Peripheral vascular—cramps, varicose veins, cold hands or feet, color or pallor
- Neurological—numbness, tingling, local weakness, memory, tremors, fainting, black-outs, seizures, paralysis
- Psychosocial—lifestyle, home situation, a typical day, important experiences, religious beliefs that may pertain to treatment or illness, perceptions of health, attitude, and outlook for future[4]

Other systems that come into play may not be adequately represented in the intake forms. For further information regarding the systems of the body and examination techniques, consult Bates' *Guide to Physical Examination* (7th edition)[4] or Magee's *Orthopaedic Physical Assessment* (2nd edition).[5]

Once you have identified symptoms—pain, stiffness, weakness, and the like—ask the client to describe the symptom's specific location, intensity, duration, frequency, and the setting in which it occurred and recurs. Record that information. For example: headache pain, pounding, left frontal, moderate minus, 2 to 3 days, monthly, with menses for 10 plus years.

Description

Once the client has identified the symptoms, ask him or her to describe them further. For example: If the symptom is pain, it may be described as sharp, shooting, dull, or aching. A client once described her numbness as "cold and wet." Record any information that qualifies the symptom and is helpful in assessing and treating it or in marking progress.

Location

Ask the client to identify the precise location of the symptom. In addition to locating the symptom, this information can be helpful in identifying the source of the dysfunction and in substantiating progress. As explained in Travell and Simons, the location of the trigger point pain can lead to proper treatment application. For example: If Moira's headache pain is located in the forehead over her right eye, the trigger point is likely to be found in the right sternocleidomastoid.[7] Progress can be demonstrated when the area of pain diminishes in size. In the story of Sandee in Chapter 2, her back pain originally covered her entire low back area. Eventually, the location of her pain was reduced to a small area around her sacrum. Be specific about the location to assist with symptom identification, assessment of the condition, and treatment application.

Intensity

Measure all symptoms by quantifying their expression. Ask clients to rate the intensity of their symptoms on a numerical scale of 0 to 10, a value scale of mild or light (L), moderate (M), and severe (S), or a descriptive scale of normal (N), good (G), fair (F), and poor (P). The value scale can stand alone as a three-point scale, or it can be extended into a nine-point scale with the addition of pluses and minuses (L–, L, L+, M–, M, M+, S–, S, S+).

Choose the rating scale that works best for you. Be consistent. If you choose a nine-point value scale, use that scale for all clients at every session.

Frequency and Duration

Note how often the symptom occurs. Use general terms like seldom, intermittent, frequent, or constant; or specific descriptions like twice a day, three times a week, or hourly to note the frequency.

Record how long the symptom lasts when it occurs. Use time to denote the duration: seconds, minutes, days, weeks, months, or years.

Onset

The onset describes the setting in which the injury or condition occurred or the external factors affecting the injury, and the date of the occurrence. Include the biomechanics of the body positions and movements involved in the injury. For example, Moira lifted a box of books from the floor to a shelf above her head. She turned to the left to pick up the box and turned to her right to set the box on the shelf.

In the case of a fall, it is important to note the body parts that came into contact with the type of surface and the order in which this occurred. Zamora, for example, was carrying a 25-pound bag of rice when she slipped on a banana peel at work. She fell backwards with her arm outstretched to break her fall, landed on a tile floor on her right hand and right hip, and ended up on her back, with her head hitting the floor and bouncing a few times. The heavy bag of rice landed on top of her. This information helps determine the treatment plan by identifying the points of impact and the angles of entry.

In the case of a repetitive movement injury, the onset includes the repeated action and a description of any other contributing data. For example: Clint hammers repeatedly at shoulder height with right hand, 20-ounce hammer, 8 hours per day, 5 days per week, 5 years at job, carrying heavy nail pouch on left hip.

Include the date of the onset. Be specific to a day, month, and year, rather than a casual reference to "since last Friday" or "when I was 16." The latter requires you to make a calculation every time you refer back to the initial SOAP note. Keep it simple.

In situations involving repetitive movement injuries, the date of the onset may be difficult to determine. As in the scenario above, help Clint determine the approximate year the symptoms began occurring. To Clint, it may feel like the pain has been going on forever, but if you prod his memory a bit by suggesting 10 years or 20 years, he's likely to giggle and remind you that he's only 23 years old and has been working construction for five years. Record a month or a time of year as well as the year of onset, if possible. Noting "Summer of '42" or "January '93" is more helpful than a simple "for many years."

Having a clear record of the mechanisms of injury will help justify treating a broader area. For example, with Moira's lift and twist injury, the diagnosis may be a low back sprain-strain. Treatment to her neck and shoulders may seem luxurious and unnecessary to a referring HCP or an insurance representative unless you can clearly explain the biomechanical links and compensating symptoms involved.

Activities of Daily Living—Aggravating and Relieving

Emphasize function, such as how well the client is able to perform daily activities, when charting subjective information. Record the client's current and prior level of function, how the symptoms affect his ability to function, and how his ability to function affects his life at home and work.

The documentation process—inquiry, discussion, and charting—increases clients' awareness of their role in exacerbating or reducing the symptoms. Record events of everyday life that aggravate or relieve symptoms to document significant injury, note progress, and educate clients to use activities that relieve rather than aggravate their symptoms.

The information regarding clients' activities of daily living will assist you in proving functional progress and providing effective self-care education. Functional limitations that have the most effect on their quality of life will be used to determine long-term and short-term goals. Use relieving activities when planning their homework and self-care regime. Goals and outcomes are documented in the Assessment section; homework is described in the Plan section.

Activities That Aggravate Symptoms

When documenting activities that aggravate the client's symptoms, be specific about home and work responsibilities, including hobbies and play activities. Generally speaking, activities involve basic functions: sitting, standing, walking, lifting, sleeping, and the like. Use the Pain Questionnaires to identify the basic functions with which clients experience difficulty. In this section of the SOAP chart, however, explain how each function personally relates to the individual's daily activities. Include the relevance of the specific activity to the client's life, how long the client can perform the activity before the symptoms begin or worsen, and compare with the client's previous ability. For example: Pain increases from mild to moderate with sitting or standing more than 30 minutes. Sits at computer 7 to 8 hours per day for work, stands in kitchen 1 to 2 hours per day doing household chores, and reads for recreation. Unable to drive comfortably for more than 10 minutes—35-mile commute to work, picks children up from day care, next week a road trip with the family through the Canyon Lands is scheduled—planned for 6 months.

Include activities the client can no longer perform because of the symptoms. For example: Unable to lift objects heavier than 25 pounds—job requires lifting objects up to 60 pounds, exercise routine included weight lifting, small children at home require lifting for care. Address endurance by describing an activity and stating the amount tolerated before signs of fatigue are exhibited. For example: Must stop reading after 20 minutes and housework after 10 minutes because of pain and fatigue.

When daily activities change noticeably but symptoms remain constant, a look at aggravating activities may reveal progress that might otherwise go undetected. Often, when clients are recovering from injuries that have limited them, the better they feel, the more they attempt to do. They are eager to return to work, get out of the house, and feel useful again. The weeds in the garden are nagging them, the stack of laundry is piling up, the kids want to get the flat tire fixed on the bike. When the activity level increases, there may be little to no improvement in symptoms—symptoms may even worsen. Rather than assuming that there is no progress, document the changes in activities. This will explain the lack of progress with the symptoms and show improvement in the client's health based on activity level.

▼

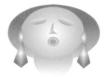

STORY TELLER
Pain Threshold Affects Client Perceptions of Progress

I was a bit lazy charting sessions with a fellow massage therapist who had been in a car collision. Angela's knee was injured in the crash and required surgery. At first, I was diligently recording her functional limitations and helping her set functional goals. For example, she was ambitious about attending the opening of a basket exhibition,

(Continued)

STORY TELLER   *(Continued)*

and we worked together to set reasonable goals regarding her ability to walk around the gallery. With frequent stops to sit and rest, she was able to see each basket in the exhibit!

Six weeks later, Angela seemed very down about her condition. She complained that she felt little progress and was experiencing pain every day while walking and standing. Realizing that weeks had gone by since I questioned her regarding her daily activities, I asked her how much walking she was doing. "I'm walking to and from work every day, and it always hurts!" I knew she lived a mile from her office atop a hill. Angela had returned to walking the two miles round trip just four weeks after her stop-and-go limp around a gallery. I was impressed! As her therapist, I was able to maintain perspective of Angela's progress, but Angela couldn't see beyond the fact that today she was in pain. Somehow, I needed to help Angela remain cognizant of her progress.

I told Angela my painful story of being introduced to 100 MDs at the CAM symposium and what I had learned from the Chronic Low Back Pain study.[8] (from the Story Teller in Chapter 1). After discussing how one's threshold of pain can affect one's perception of progress, she agreed that we had not focused adequately on her functional successes; namely, the dramatic shift in her ability to walk. We made a commitment to set goals every month and regularly evaluate her functional progress until all her goals for health were met.

Activities That Relieve Symptoms

List activities that alleviate symptoms. Include modifying necessary activities, self-care, exercises, or remedies that relieve the symptoms. Changing positions, taking frequent breaks, stretching exercises, self-massage, topical analgesics, and hot or cold packs are also considered activities that alleviate symptoms.

Investigate closely the steps the client has taken to care for herself. Uncover as many ways as possible that the client participates in her health care. Document specific activities that you want to reinforce or that have been particularly effective. For example: Catherine Ann applies ice to low back as needed for pain, sits on a tennis ball to relieve trigger point pain, and squeezes tennis ball throughout day to exercise hands. You may choose not to record all the information uncovered, but use it to compliment the client, build her self-esteem, and encourage her to continue to participate in her health care.

OBJECTIVE

This section of the SOAP chart stores information from the practitioner's perspective:

◆   Measurable data—movement tests, palpatory findings, visual observations
◆   Treatment applications—techniques, location, duration
◆   Client's response to the massage

State information clearly and concisely. Stick to details within your scope of practice. Do not chart treatment techniques for which you cannot explain the physiological effects clearly and consistently. Avoid data that cannot be measured or reproduced.

Massage therapists primarily gather the following objective, measurable data: visual observations, such as posture and breath; palpatory findings, such as spasms and trigger points; movement and strength tests, such as gait analysis and active, passive, and resistive ROM tests. Document all tests uniformly and consistently.

Follow these simple guidelines when gathering and charting your objective findings:

◆ Document a full range of data.
◆ Measure every finding.
◆ Measure before and after treatment application.
◆ Perform the post-assessment in the same way as the pre-assessment.
◆ Use consistent terminology and symbols.

The data you record should represent the full scope of your practice. Do not limit yourself by narrowly focusing on one aspect of your expertise. This can cause problems when others in your profession exercise the full extent of the professional scope.

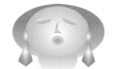

STORY TELLER
The Laundry List of Hypertonicities

I attended a meeting with reviewers and medical directors from a few insurance companies. I was there to defend the scope of practice of massage therapists as a result of a narrowing interpretation of our assessment and treatment abilities. The medical director of one of the health plans claimed she was getting hypertonicities from reading about all the hypertonicities on therapists' SOAP charts. She wanted to know why the providers in her network insisted on listing every tight muscle in the body and nothing else, and whether indeed the therapists were capable of noting inflammation, spasms, trigger points, joint dysfunction, and such. Tight muscles alone do not provide a convincing argument for medical necessity. Balance your objective charting by noting a variety of findings.

Measure all information. Quantify and qualify data based on deviations from normal. Normal is determined by:

◆ Comparing bilaterally when possible
◆ Defining normal for a general population of similar constitution
◆ Asking the client to define normal for himself or herself

Quantify data by rating the intensity of its expression. For example: trigger point moderately painful with light digital pressure at the trigger point site and mildly painful at the referral site; or, cervical flexion passive range of motion was limited 4/10 with 2/10 pain at end range.

Qualify data by describing its expression. For example: right shoulder active abduction moderate segmented movement with mild compensatory shoulder elevation at end range; or, moderate plus sharp shooting pain with movement from prone to supine position while turning on treatment table.

Assess the condition before and after treatment. It is difficult to document progress or determine the effectiveness of a treatment modality without being able to do a before-and-after comparison. For example: moderate trigger point site pain changed to mild pain, mild referred pain changed to no pain; or, moderate segmented movement in right shoulder active abduction changed to smooth movement without compensatory shoulder elevation.

Perform tests identically for pre-treatment and post-treatment. Data must be comparable. For example, postural analysis in a standing position (weight bearing) provides different information from postural analysis in a supine or seated position (non-weight bearing). Therefore, the client should be in the same position for both tests. Also, reproduce the test in the original environment. For example: If the client was sitting in a chair for the pre-treatment range of motion assessment, he should be sitting in the same chair, not on the treatment table, for the post-treatment assessment.

Be consistent from session to session. It is difficult to compare data over time when the range of motion testing was done standing initially, seated last session, and supine this session. Also, take into consideration the timing of the tests. If the initial test was done on a Friday afternoon after a long week at work, and the test was reassessed on a Monday morning after a relaxing weekend, the data will not be comparable.

Pick qualifying and quantifying terms and use them consistently. Smooth, segmented, and spastic may describe the quality of the range of motion. Sharp and dull can be used to qualify pain. Numerical scales (0 to 10) or value scales (L, M, S) can quantify data. Select terms that adequately represent your assessment test results. Create abbreviations for the terms when necessary and add them to your legend. Most importantly, use the same terms consistently from session to session and client to client.

Visual Observations

Visual findings stem from observing movement patterns such as posture, muscle atrophy, skin abnormalities, swelling, and signs of trauma (such as bruises, abrasions, and scars). Much of the visual data can be recorded on the SOAP chart by drawing symbols on the human figures. For example: Posture is easily noted on the figures by drawing skewed lines to depict elevations and arrows in the direction of rotations. Use standard symbols to represent visual findings, or you may add your own to the key. Functional movement patterns, such as gait or respiration, and comments about general appearance are more easily noted in the space provided for written information (see Figure 5-2).

Follow these guidelines for documenting posture and movement patterns:

◆ Note the position of the client—seated, standing, prone, supine
◆ Record the angle of the observation—anterior, lateral, posterior
◆ Describe the activity being observed—breathing, walking, lifting, standing
◆ Follow the guidelines for gathering and charting objective findings (listed previously)

For example: client supine, anterior-lateral view, deep inhalation, mild plus mobility restriction upper right quadrant.

Posture can be quantified by rating the amount of deviation from normal. Simply mark a number or letter denoting the intensity of the deviation near the line or arrow as it is drawn on the figures.

FIGURE 5–2 Objective: Visual and palpable observations

John Olson, LMP, GCFP
345 Moon River Rd. Ste. 6
Minnehaha, MN   55987
TEL   612 555 9889

HANDS HEAL

SOAP CHART-M

Client Name   _Darnel G. Washington_   Date _2-6-04_

Date of Injury _1-6-04_   ID#/DOB _123-45-6789_ Meds _hydrocodone 500mg q4h_

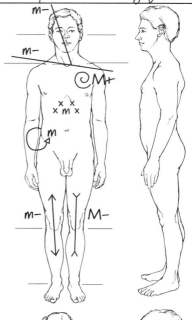

O   Findings: Visual/Palpable/Test Results

v: Primary weight bearing rising and standing-
    right leg and foot-moderate
    sits on right pelvis-moderate
    bends from mid-thoracic-moderate
    breath shallow and rapid-moderate
    segmental rib movement on left with deep inhalation-
        moderate

P: right frontal torsion-moderate
    bilateral sphenoid compression-moderate
    adhesion tentorium-mild
    cranial rhythm weak, right-moderate
        left-mild

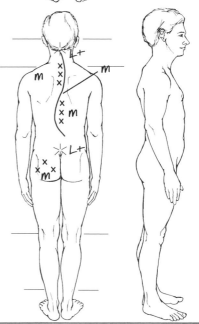

Therapist's Signature _JO, LMP, GCFP_   Date _2-6-04_

Legend:

℮ TP	• TeP	○ ℗	✳ Infl	≡ HT	≈ SP
✕ Adh	≷ Numb	◯ rot	╱ elev	⊶ Short	⟷ Long

87

Chart irregularities: forward head posture, leg length variations, spinal curvatures, and the like. Note elevations, rotations, inversions, and eversions. Common sites for observing posture are at the ears, shoulders, superior and inferior angles of the scapulae, anterior and posterior superior iliac spine, knees, and the medial and lateral malleoli.

Breath can be measured by qualifying the pattern and rate of breath, describing sounds associated with breathing, and quantifying the mobility of the ribs with inhalation. Note irregularities such as a rattling noise or shallow, rapid, weak, uneven, or inconsistent patterns in breathing. Observe the rise and fall of the ribs and chart the restrictions.

Functional movement patterns can be qualified and quantified by noting the amount of movement, how well the movement is performed, and how long the client can sustain the movement before experiencing fatigue. Note sensations caused by movement and rate their expression.

Palpation Findings

Palpation is an objective test used to locate and assess inconsistencies in various rhythms, pulses, and systems of the body such as soft tissue, joints, viscera, and lymph. Massage therapists tend to be highly trained and adept at sensing subtle discrepancies and changes under their fingers. As a result, detailed palpatory information is a valuable resource for all caregivers involved in the client's health care team, and the information can be shared through SOAP charts and progress reports.

Document palpation findings by noting and describing abnormalities and conditions. Terminology varies among professions and specialties. Compile a comprehensive list of evaluative terms for your practice and use the terms consistently. Your list may include:

- Muscle tone—including tension, hypertonic, hypotonic, spastic, rigid, splinting, contracture, spasm, lines of tension, holding patterns
- Pain—including trigger points, tender points, meridian points, Jones points, absence of sensation, spasm-pain-spasm cycle. (Note: Pain is usually considered subjective information. Pain becomes objective when it is elicited by the practitioner through touch, testing, etc.)
- Scar tissue—adhesions, fibrosis, fibrotic tissue, granulation tissue
- Inflammation—including swelling, edema, active hyperemia, ischemia, congestion, stagnation, heat, pitted edema

Avoid diagnostic terms—such as Grade II sprain or strain and lymphedema—to describe findings if you do not have diagnostic scope or if the referring HCP or the client did not provide you with diagnostic information.

Measure the palpation data by rating the intensity of the finding, such as with severe spasm, or quantifying the size, such as with right ankle edema 20 centimeters in circumference.

Much of the data collected through palpation is documented easily on human figures using symbols found in the legend. Write the quantifying or qualifying terms next to the figure. Whenever necessary, tie the letter or number to the symbol with a connecting line. Anything too complicated or cumbersome to draw on the figures can be written out in the space provided (refer to Figure 5-2). The figures are intended to increase the speed and ease of documentation and to aid in fast recall. This intent is defeated if the figures are overburdened with symbols. When the data are abundant, draw the primary information on the figures and list the secondary data in the space provided under Objective.

Follow these guidelines when documenting palpation findings:

◆ Identify the specific location.
◆ Rate or describe the type of touch that triggers the finding (for example: light, medium, or deep).
◆ Include any referred sensation, if applicable.
◆ Identify connections or relationships, if any.
◆ Follow the guidelines for gathering and charting objective findings (listed earlier in this chapter).

For example: left biceps insertion moderate pain with light digital pressure, mild plus referred pain into left elbow.

Range of Motion Testing

The most common standardized testing for massage therapists is **range of motion (ROM)** testing (see forms in Appendix: Blank Forms). It is used in many professions and is familiar to lay people as a means of assessing health. A popular television commercial shows a person bending over and touching his toes, at first with limitation and pain, then—after taking the product—with greater range and ease. The message: Greater movement with less discomfort equals better health. As a result, many clients expect ROM testing from any practitioner assessing and treating joint pain.

range of motion: a movement test to access the available motion allowed by the shape of the joint and the soft tissue surrounding it

ROM testing is a valuable assessment tool for determining the stage of inflammation, the level of severity of sprains and strains, joint trauma, and muscle weakness. Gather and record ROM test results to substantiate dysfunction, validate progress, and identify conditions. Assessing ROM before treatment substantiates the limitations for the client. Retesting ROM after intervention demonstrates the effectiveness of the treatment plan and proves progress resulting from the session. Periodic testing at pre-treatment and post-treatment times shows continued progress and gives the client, the referring caregivers, and the insurance reviewers evidence that the treatment is working.

Document the test:

◆ Identify the position of the client—standing, seated, prone, supine, sidelying
◆ Identify the type of test—active, active assisted, passive, resistive
◆ Name the joint—including right shoulder, left hip, cervical spine
◆ Name the action—including flexion, extension, left rotation, right lateral flexion

Chart the results of the test (see Figure 5-3):

◆ Rate the amount of movement as a deviation from normal—hypermobile, hypomobile, within normal limits (for example: moderate decrease in seated active cervical flexion . . .)
◆ Rate the presense of pain with movement or stretch (for example: . . . with moderate pain.)
◆ Rate the quality of the movement—including smooth, segmented, spastic, rigid (for example: . . . with mild segmented movement.)

ROM test results are commonly expressed in degrees or percentages of normal. If you are not using measuring devices such as goniometers, use the numerical scale of 0 to 10 or the value scale of mild, moderate, and severe to rate ROM test results. You will be able to show deviations from normal with enough detail to note progress as changes develop. (For information on how to perform ROM tests or use goniometric measurements, see Kendall et al.[9] or Norkin and White.[10])

Treatment

Document the length of the session, the massage techniques and modalities used, and the location of the treatments that were applied. Record the treatment in two ways. First, provide a big picture of the session—the length of the session, techniques, and general body parts treated. For example: 1-hour full-body Swedish massage; 30-minute foot reflexology; or 90-minute Hellerwork—inspiration. Second, fill in the details—particular techniques used to treat specific findings. For example: muscle energy technique with cervical flexion, direct pressure on scalene trigger point, or myofascial release on diaphragm. You do not need to write down everything you do; just give the highlights. Chart enough information to recall the important events of the session at a later date.

Client's Response to Treatment

Every subjective and objective finding should be reassessed during the session. This may happen as you go—immediately after a specific technique is applied to address a particular symptom—or at the end of the session.

Quantify and qualify the changes. Include positive and negative responses to treatment. Record the updated information on the chart above or alongside the original entry. Use the delta symbol (Δ) to distinguish the pre-treatment data from the post-treatment entry (see Figure 5-4). This is an efficient way to document the client's response and avoid rewriting in several places on the chart.

FIGURE 5–3 ROM Chart

John Olson, LMP, GCFP
345 Moon River Rd. Ste. 6
Minnehaha, MN   55987
HANDS HEAL   TEL   612 555 9889

RANGE OF MOTION

Client Name __Darnel G. Washington__   Date __2-6-04__

Date of Injury __1-6-04__   ID#/DOB __123-45-6789__

PRE-TEST 1 Initials __JO__   Date __2-6-04__

Position of patient: prone, sidelying, sitting, (standing,) supine, other: _____

Type of test: (active,) active assisted, passive, resistive, other: _____

Joint: C-spine, T-spine, (L-spine,) hip, knee, ankle, shoulder, elbow, wrist, other: _____

Action	Quantify ↓ or ↑		Rate Pain		Rate Quality	
	(R)	(L)	(R)	(L)	(R)	(L)
flex	M⁻	↓	L⁺		L	seg
ext	M⁺	↓	M		M	seg
SB	L↓	M↓	L	M	N	Mseg

POST-TEST 1 Initials __JO__   Date __2-6-04__

Position of patient: prone, sidelying, sitting, (standing,) supine, other: _____

Type of test: (active,) active assisted, passive, resistive, other: _____

Joint: C-spine, T-spine, (L-spine,) hip, knee, ankle, shoulder, elbow, wrist, other: _____

Action	Quantify ↓ or ↑		Rate Pain		Rate Quality	
	(R)	(L)	(R)	(L)	(R)	(L)
flex	L	↓	0		N	
ext	M	↓	M⁺		L	seg
SB	X	X	X	L	N	L seg

FIGURE 5–4 Objective: Response to treatment

John Olson, LMP, GCFP
345 Moon River Rd. Ste. 6
Minnehaha, MN   55987
HANDS HEAL   TEL 612 555 9889

SOAP CHART-M

Client Name _Darnel G. Washington_   Date _2-6-04_

Date of Injury _1-6-04_   ID#/DOB _123-45-6789_ Meds _hydrocodone 500mg_   ℞

S   Symptoms: Location/Intensity/Frequency/Duration/Onset

Neck, mid, low back pain moderate
constant since car accident △ L
headache Pain moderate intermittant
daily since car accident △ ℗

O   Findings: Visual/Palpable/Test Results

Primary weight bearing rising and standing
right leg and   oot-moderate⊠
sits on right pel   is-moderate⊠
bends   rom mid-thoracic-moderate△ L
breath shallow and rapid-moderate △ L
segmental rib mo   ement on le   t with deep inhalation-
      moderate △ smooth
P   right   rontal torsion-modera△ L
bilateral sphenoid compression-moderate △   –
adhesion tentori   m-milc⊠
cranial rhythm weak, right-moderate △ L
      le   t-milo△ Normal

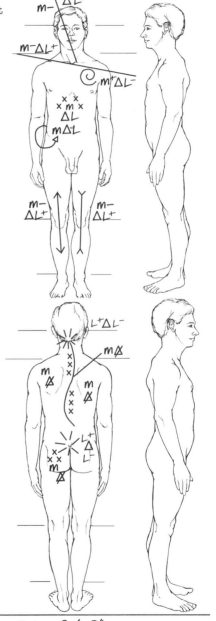

Therapist's Signature _____, L P, G   P_____   Date _2-6-04_

Legend: ℮ TP   • TeP   ○ ℗   ✳ Infl   ≡ HT   ≈ SP
                 ✕ Adh   ≋ Numb   ⟲ rot   ╱ elev   ⊶ Short   ⟷ Long

Note symptoms and measurable data that did not change. This may help you determine areas of focus for the next session. Identify whether the treatment was ineffective or that time did not permit addressing the issue. In either case, you will want to address the problem in the treatment plan; make the issue a priority for the next session or select another technique to use. "No change" is easily abbreviated with a line drawn through the delta symbol. (Δ̸)

ASSESSMENT

Traditionally, the Assessment section of the SOAP chart records the practitioner's interpretation of the subjective and objective findings. Conclusions are drawn, the condition is named (diagnosis), and the prognosis—probable course of the disease—is determined and recorded on the SOAP chart. However, practitioners without diagnostic scope are not permitted to assess the client's condition in these terms.

In functional outcomes reporting, assessment is the place to summarize the client's functional ability—to set goals that, when accomplished, demonstrate functional progress. Every practitioner using the functional approach to SOAP charting will record functional goals and outcomes in the Assessment section. If the client does not have any functional limitations, but does have a medical condition that warrants SOAP charting, leave this section blank. Before you fall back on this option, however, question the client regarding his or her sleep patterns. Most people living with pain have disruptions in their sleep, even when they are still able to perform all other activities of daily living without modification. If they are waking during the night because of pain or are waking in the morning feeling fatigued, set measurable goals regarding sleep and note measurable progress as they achieve their goals.

Record the following under Assessment:

◆ Long-term and short-term functional goals based in activities of daily living
◆ Functional outcomes

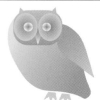

WISE ONE SPEAKS
Follow the Client's Lead

"You should never have expectations for other people. . . . setting goals for others can be aggressive—really wanting a success story for ourselves. When we do this to others, we are asking them to live up to our ideals. Instead, just be kind."[11] This quote from Trungpa Rinpoche reminds us to follow the client's lead in setting goals. Remember that the client is in charge in the therapeutic relationship. SOAP notes were designed to help formulate a high-quality treatment plan and promote the practitioner's problem-solving skills. This same format can be equally effective in promoting the client's problem-solving skills by adding the functional outcomes approach to our information gathering and charting. Focus on the therapeutic relationship and prioritize the client's goals above our own in every step of SOAP charting.

The functional outcomes style of documentation is increasingly popular and benefits the client, the practitioner, and all who read the chart because it directly addresses the basic needs of the client, monitors effective treatment, and makes the results easily understood—not just to the experts.

Functional Outcomes Begin as Goals

Functional outcomes are written in the form of functional goals, set by the client with practitioner guidance. Goals are determined through the activities with which the client is having difficulty and with which the client is motivated to resume. As they are accomplished, the goals are identified as functional outcomes.

Develop goals that address the needs of the client and lead to an effective treatment plan—one that will resolve the client's concerns. With the client, follow these steps:

◆ Summarize and prioritize verbally the client's functional limitations, referring to what is already written in the Subjective section of the SOAP chart.
◆ Relate these functional limitations to all meaningful and pertinent activities of daily living (ADLs) and review these with the client.
◆ Select one activity that is adversely affected by the client's condition—one to which the client is most motivated to return.
◆ Create and record long-term and short-term SMART goals (LTG, STG) based on that ADL.

Setting SMART Goals

To ensure that the goals will lead to productive treatment plans and produce functional outcomes that serve the client's needs, follow the **SMART goals** criteria.[12] The acronym SMART stands for the following:

Specific—to a daily activity

Measurable—quantified and qualified to note incremental progress

Attainable—able to be accomplished given the client's condition

Relevant—critical to the client's daily life

Time-bound—defined to be successful in a specific amount of time

With the client, build functional goals that meet the SMART criteria.

SMART goals: acronym for Specific, Measurable, Attainable, Relevant, Time-bound; a system for creating well-defined functional goals

SMART—Specific and Relevant Activity

Select activities that are specific and functional. This can include vacuuming, mowing the lawn, washing hair, lifting boxes onto a conveyor belt, loading and unloading furniture to a truck, rowing a boat, and the like. The more specific the activity, the better. "Work," "exercise," "child care," and "housework" are not specific enough to base a functional goal on. If house cleaning is the work, explore the activity that increases the symptoms—is it standing at the sink, pushing a vacuum cleaner, pulling sheets off a bed, lifting laundry, scrubbing floors? If computer programming is the work, is it sitting still, staring at the screen, moving the mouse? If the exercise is playing tennis, is it the forehand stroke, backhand, serve, lateral moves? What part of child care is problematic—lifting the child, leaning over to play with her, picking up the toys?

Reducing pain is a common goal of the client, but is not functional—based on an activity. Pain is a qualifier, measuring the success of a goal. If a client states "pain free" as his goal, guide him to a specific activity by exploring activities that cause the pain.

Select the activity that is most relevant to the client's life. Address work, home, family, exercise, and play activities. The goal should be based on an activity that is critical to the client's ability to earn a living or care for himself, his family, or his household. If the injury occurred on the job and industrial insurance is paying for the treatment, select a work-related activity.

SMART—Measurable and Time-bound

Once the specific and relevant activity is selected, specify how the success of the goal will be gauged.

1. Quantify the outcome by measuring the activity—number of units, amount of weight, repetitions, duration, or frequency
2. Qualify the outcome by projecting how the client will feel upon completion—amount of pain, fatigue, or functional limitations
3. Schedule a time limit for completion—commonly 30 to 60 days for LTG or about 1 to 2 weeks for STG. Be specific: 45 days, not 30 to 60 days

   For example: Lift 25-pound boxes from a three-foot-high, moving conveyor belt and stack them onto hand trucks for 30 minutes keeping pace with the conveyor with no more than mild pain within six weeks.

1. Quantify the outcome—Lift 25-pound boxes from a three-foot-high, moving conveyor belt and stack them onto hand trucks for 30 minutes keeping pace with the conveyor
2. Qualify the outcome—with no more than mild pain
3. Time-bound—within six weeks

   Climb up and down four standard steps at a moderate pace three times a day with moderate pain and mild fatigue within one week.

1. Quantify the outcome—Climb up and down four standard steps at a moderate pace three times a day
2. Qualify the outcome—with moderate pain and mild fatigue
3. Time-bound—within one week

   Sleep restfully for three hours without waking once each night with mild fatigue upon waking within two weeks

1. Quantify the outcome—Sleep restfully for three hours without waking once each night
2. Qualify the outcome—with mild fatigue upon waking
3. Time-bound—within two weeks

   Two standard time frames can be used: long-term and short-term. LTGs are developed first. Identify the desired end result of the treatment. If it is not possible to reach the goal in 30 to 60 days, write one or two intermediary LTGs, each one attainable within 30 to 60 days.

   STGs are established to support the LTG and are often written as incremental stages of the LTG. Think of them as baby steps toward the end result. If the end result is to lift boxes up to 50-pounds from the floor to a truck up to 100 times a day for five days a week, write STGs that are fractions of the original goal. For example:

   STG #1: Lift 10 pounds from a three-foot-high shelf 10 times a day within 12 days

   STG #2: Lift 20 pounds from a two-foot-high shelf 10 times, two times a day within 20 days

   STG #3: Lift 30 pounds from a one-foot-high shelf 20 times, three times a day within 12 days

Write STGs that provide encouragement and motivation for the client, even if the STG does not appear to be directly related to the original goal. For example: LTG—pain free and fully functional while swimming the breast stroke for 1,500 meters within 30 days. If the breast stroke is painful because of a neck injury but the client is eager to experience success in the water, set a goal that provides a feeling of success in the water. STG—one-week goal of 30 minutes of water aerobics with moderate pain. The aerobic exercises may not require the client to extend her neck—the function that causes her pain—and being in the water may be very comforting for her. The result is an immediate feeling of accomplishment that may not be realized with long-term goals.

The time limit for LTGs is often dictated by the prescription length. One or two STGs should be written for each LTG. Determine the measurements for the time frames by assessing the possibilities for each client, given his or her condition and constitution.

SMART—Attainable

Be reasonable when writing goals. A goal that is too vast—pain free and fully functional while swimming the breast stroke for 1,500 meters within 30 days—can be frustrating to reach when the client is currently unable to swim at all. If we are to eliminate the client's feelings of powerlessness and inspire her to work hard to achieve her goals, we must develop goals that are not only meaningful but continually are within her reach. Evaluate the severity of the injury, the client's constitution, and functional status, then determine whether the goal as stated is attainable for the client in the allotted time.

It is helpful to pre-determine how the client's body will respond to treatment. Don't worry if you misjudge this; you can adjust the goal at the following session by renegotiating the time limit or the outcome measurements. Instead of swimming 1,500 meters with no pain, adjust the outcome to:

The client will be able to swim 500 meters with moderate pain within 30 days.

PLAN

The Plan section charts the future treatment protocol and records self-care exercises. Set treatment goals and list probable treatment options for obtaining the goals. Outline the frequency of the sessions and duration of each and settle on an approximate reevaluation date. Chart specific instructions for homework suggestions. Document your referrals and recommendations for outside interventions and tests.

Treatment Plan

The initial note projects the plans for the first series of treatments. First, given the information shared in the extensive initial interview and full-body assessment, determine and prioritize your goals for the series:

1. Reduce inflammation in the neck
2. Reduce pain in the neck and shoulders
3. Increase ROM of the neck

Next, the practitioner and the client select massage techniques and modalities to employ that will accomplish your goals and the client's functional goals. Base your decision about treatment techniques on what has worked for the client in the past and what has worked for others who have had similar conditions and constitution. List the techniques projected and the general locations for applying the massage. For example:

1. Lymphatic drainage and ice packs on the neck to reduce the inflammation
2. Swedish massage and trigger point therapy on the neck and shoulders to reduce pain
3. Muscle energy technique to the levator scapulae and sternocleidomastoid to increase ROM

Record the frequency of the subsequent sessions—3 times a week, weekly, or monthly; duration of sessions—30 minutes, 1 hour, 90 minutes; and the reevaluation date. The plan should cover the length of the prescription or the time allotted for the LTG. If you are treating the client twice a week, a 30-day reevaluation date is appropriate. If the treatment frequency is once a week, 45 days between reevaluations may feel adequate. For example: 45-minute sessions, twice a week for three weeks; reevaluation during week of 6-15-04.

Update the plan every 30 days or more, depending on the treatment frequency. Modify the plan more frequently whenever the client's condition changes or the plan is no longer appropriate based on the client's response to the previous treatments. Let the treatment plan guide you, but do not let it dictate the sessions. Be flexible and respond to individual needs as they arise. Remain mindful of the goals at the same time.

Self-Care

self-care: the client's active participation in the healing process. Includes remedial exercise, hydro-therapy, self-message, diaphragmatic breathing, and referrals to other practitioners, self-help groups, or exercise programs.

Record **self-care** exercises and homework assignments that support the goals. Self-care is a broad term that includes modifying activities to decrease pain and effort and increase safety, stretching and strengthening exercises, and home remedies such as ice packs, Epson salt baths, polstices, ointments, and self-massage techniques. Compliment the client on everything he currently does to improve his condition and reinforce his efforts by charting the self-care exercises that are most productive.

Be specific and provide detailed instructions when assigning homework. Support the client's self-care routine by recording the homework assignment and the specific instructions or attaching a copy of the instruction sheet to the chart. This is difficult to do if we cannot remember the assignment. For example: Stand up and stretch for two minutes for every hour of work at the computer. Hold all stretches for 30 seconds. Stretches include

bending over slowly and touching toes, return to standing
bending over to each side, return to standing
pulling arms behind back using filing cabinet; before sitting down, walk to the water fountain and drink

Keep homework simple. Make sure it fits into the client's lifestyle. If the client is very busy, homework should not be too time-consuming. New exercises should not be too complex, so assign activities the client will find familiar and comfortable. Ideally, homework should be the client's idea or a modification of something the client suggests.

Remember, do not provide homework to people who are not ready for it. Some clients do not yet believe that change is possible. Assign awareness exercises for clients who are unaware of their role in the healing process and don't seem to recognize change when it occurs. Invite them to notice the way they feel when they are performing an activity that exacerbates their condition. For example: For every hour spent at the computer, stop and take a break. Notice how your neck, back, arms, and hands feel. Notice whether anything you do makes that feeling better or worse.

Initial Notes, Subsequent Notes, Progress Notes, and Discharge Notes

Four types of notes are recorded on the two SOAP formats: the extended version and the sort version. The extended version is a full-page SOAP chart with multiple prompting categories. The short version is a half-page form with only the SOAP sections noted (see forms in Appendix: Blank Forms).

◆ Initial notes (extended version)
◆ Subsequent notes (short version)
◆ Progress notes (extended version)
◆ Discharge notes (extended version)

The initial notes are comprehensive and include extensive information regarding the client's health and current situation. Much of the information recorded on an initial SOAP chart does not need to be repeated on subsequent notes.

◆ List and prioritize all the client's health concerns.
◆ Evaluate the full body, including the way the client is responding to his or her current health situation from head to toe.
◆ Include all symptoms that relate to the client's health concerns, the impact of the condition on the client's life, and all objective findings, including compensational holding patterns and concomitant dysfunctions.
◆ Discuss and create functional goals—after the initial assessment and treatment—that can be used as a measurement of the success of the relationship in language to which the client can relate.
◆ Determine the treatment plan that will best address the needs of the client and move toward accomplishing the goals.
◆ Use the extended version of the SOAP form (see Figure 5-5).

Subsequent SOAP notes are brief and primarily record the treatment provided. The focus is on the client's immediate presenting concerns with consideration to the proposed treatment plan. The notes are less comprehensive in regards to assessment and are more specific to the data directly related to the treatment provided. For example: On Darnel's initial SOAP chart, all cervical actions and ranges of motion were tested and recorded. On a subsequent note in which the focus of treatment was to decrease neck stiffness, only the cervical active range of motion for lateral flexion was tested, charted, treated, and retested. The intent is to spend more time accomplishing goals than assessing the condition and determining the plan. The treatment plan is projected initially and reviewed during reevaluation sessions. Subsequent sessions carry out the treatment plan. The chart should reflect that and not repeat the goals or treatment plans unless changes are necessary. Often, the Assessment and Plan sections of the SOAP chart are left blank on subsequent notes. The Assessment section should only reflect functional outcomes or changes to the goals. The Plan section in a subsequent note need only chart additional homework assignments or self-care education, unless the treatment plan needs to be altered. A shorter version of the initial SOAP form is adequate for recording information between the initial visit and the reevaluation sessions (see Figure 5-6).

Progress SOAP notes are used to chart reevaluation sessions. Reevaluation sessions are nearly as extensive as initial visits. Time is spent assessing progress, setting new goals,

subsequent SOAP notes: brief notes addressing the patient's immediate concerns for the day's session

progress SOAP notes: comprehensive notes for recording reevaluation and reexamination sessions

FIGURE 5-5 Initial SOAP Chart

HANDS HEAL

John Olson, LMP, GCFP
345 Moon River Rd. Ste. 6
Minnehaha, MN   55987
Tel   612 555 9889

SOAP CHART-M

Client Name   _Darnel G. Washington_   Date _2-6-04_

Date of Injury _1-6-04_   ID#/DOB _123-45-6789_ Meds _hydrocodone 500mg_   Ħ

S   Focus for Today   ↓ Pain in head, neck, back

   Symptoms: Location/Intensity/Frequency/Duration/Onset
   Neck, midback, low back pain moderate
   constant since car accident △ L
   headache Pain moderate intermittant
   daily since car accident △ Ⓟ

   Activities of Daily Living: Aggravating/Relieving
      1. li ting grandda ghter necessary or care in o t o car seat, high
      chair, bed etc. Ⓟ M+ pain e ery tim
   2. gardening egetable and lower garden, bonding time with wi e nable
      to garden o er 5 min.
   3. nable to sit play bridge o er 30 min.
         rest, heat

O   Findings: Visual/Palpable/Test Results
      Primary weight bearing rising and standing-
      right leg and oot△
      sits on right pel is△ Ll balance
      bends rom mid thoracic△
      breath moderately shallow and rapid △ L e en
      mild to moderate segmental mo ement le t ribs
         with deep inhalation △ smooth
   P moderate right rontal torsion△ L
      moderate pl s bilateral sphenoid compression△ M⁻
      mild pl s adhesion tentori △
      cranial rhythm moderately weak right △ L
      mild le t△ Normal
   Modalities: Applications/Locations
   97140 Lymph Drainage tr nk
   60 min. Craniosacral-head
         Feldenkrais eyes and eet
   Response to Treatment see △

A   oals: Long term/Short term
   L G L i t grandda ghter at least 10 times per day rom the loor and
         carry her or 10 min tes with mild pain and atig e 5 days pe
         week in 60 days
         G L i t light weight toys rom loor 10 times per day 3 days per
         week in 2 weeks with mild pain
   Functional Outcomes

P   Future Treatment/Frequency
   2 times per week or 3 weeks, 60 min. sessions, contin e with lymph
   drainage, craniosacral and Feldenkrais, oc s on ribs, diaphragms, increase
   mobility and decrease adhesions
   Home or /Self care
   contin e sing heat on mid back b t a oid it on neck and low back
   switch to ice. Deep breathing e ercise

Provider Signature   _JO, LMP, GCFP_   Date _2-6-04_

Legend: ℮ TP   ● TeP   ○ Ⓟ   ✳ Infl   ≡ HT   ≈ SP
          ✕ Adh   ≋ Numb   ⟲ rot   ╱ elev   ⊷ Short   ↔ Long

FIGURE 5-6 Subsequent SOAP Chart

John Olson, LMP, GCFP
345 Moon River Rd. Ste. 6
Minnehaha, MN   55987
TEL   612 555 9889

HANDS HEAL

SOAP CHART-M

Client Name ___Darnel G. Washington___   Date __2-8-04__

Date of Injury __1-6-04__   ID#/DOB __123-45-6789__ Meds __hydrocodone 500mg q4h__

S   Focus-decrease pain in head and neck

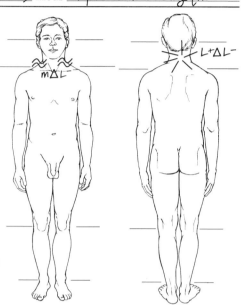

O   97140   60 min
Lymph Drainage neck, head

A   F.O.-lifting lightweight toys from shelves with
moderate pain

P   having good success with ice and breathing exercises
con't as instructed

Therapist's Signature __JO LMP GCFP__   Date ___2-8-04___

S   Focus-decrease pain in head & neck

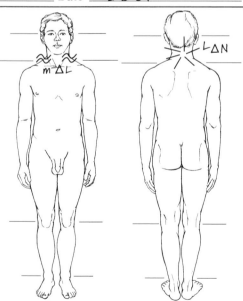

O   97140 60 min
Lymph Drainage neck, head, chest, arms,
all passive cervical ranges of motion limited-mild
minus-with mild pain at end ranges Δ N
with L⁻ pain

A   con't

P   con't

Therapist's Signature __JO LMP GCFP__   Date ___2-11-04___

Legend: ℮ TP   • TeP   ○ ℗   ✳ Infl   ≡ HT   ≈ SP
              ✕ Adh   ≋ Numb   ↺ rot   ╱ elev   ⊱ Short   ↔ Long

99

and creating new treatment plans. Schedule reevaluation sessions at every 6 to 8 visits and document them thoroughly. The notes for these sessions should be comprehensive and include a full-body evaluation.

Address everything mentioned in the initial note. There is no need to introduce new assessment tests unless new symptoms arise. It is critical, however, to revisit all previous assessments, even if the corresponding symptoms are no longer an issue. The intent is to put to rest some data and to measure the progress of the remaining data. For example: Initially, Darnel had moderate, constant, low back pain; moderate, frequent headaches; and mild, constant neck stiffness. Thirty days later, in the first progress note, Darnel reported moderate, constant, low back pain; mild, intermittant headaches; but no neck stiffness (It is important to record the fact that there is no neck stiffness). Without a record of that information, one could question whether the neck stiffness was resolved or whether or not the practitioner simply forgot to note its existence. Once a symptom or objective finding is noted as a non-issue, it does not need to be revisited in any future progress note unless the symptom or finding returns.

The intent of the progress note is to present a complete, current picture of the client's health. A comparison of the initial note and a progess note (or two consecutive progress notes) will provide summary information for **progress reports**, which are typed on letterhead stationary and sent as a courtesy to referring the HCP. Progress notes are recorded on the extended version of a SOAP form and are similar to the initial SOAP chart (see Figure 5-7).

progress reports: summary of the patient's progess and suggested additions or changes to the treatment plan submitted in letter format to the referring HCP every 30 days

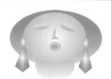

STORY TELLER
Assessment IS Treatment

A manual therapist in the Bay Area conducted a case study of all her patients to investigate the impact of information gathering on the patients' health. In every session over a one-year span, she began with range of motion testing. After recording the results, she continued to gather data, inquire about how patients felt and how their lives were impacted by the symptoms, and record postural and palpation findings. After 10 minutes of information gathering, she repeated the range of motion test. Surprisingly, the simple act of observing and recording patients' concerns resulted in a 50% improvement, on average, in range of motion. As the therapist, it is important to believe that the treatment time is well spent. This statistic may also convince patients—who are reluctant to take time away from the hands-on portion of the session—of the importance of information gathering and charting.

discharge SOAP notes: final summary of the patient's progress, health status, and subsequent course of action to be taken

Upon completion of the therapeutic relationship or when the transition is made from treatment massage to wellness care, **discharge SOAP notes** are recorded. These include a final summary of the client's progress, health status, and any subsequent course of action. Use the same SOAP form you used for the progress notes and adapt the Plan section to cover discharge data. Write the reasons for discharge, such as sessions reached limits of referral, client met goals for care, or client reached plateau in progress, in place of the treatment plan. Ongoing care may be required to maintain the progress established. Document any further action to be taken by the client. Record the self-care regimen you recommend,

FIGURE 5–7 Progress SOAP chart with discharge plan

John Olson, LMP, GCFP
345 Moon River Rd. Ste. 6
Minnehaha, MN   55987
TEL   612 555 9889

HANDS HEAL

SOAP CHART-M

Client Name   _Darnel G. Washington_   Date _1-20-05_

Date of Injury _1-6-04_   ID#/DOB _123-45-6789_ Meds   _∅_

S   Focus for Today   _decrease stiffback_

Symptoms: Location/Intensity/Frequency/Duration/Onset

_Stiff mid back mild constant for 4 days since bridge marathon
last weekend Δ within normal limits_

Activities of Daily Living: Aggravating/Relieving

_carrying granddaughter more than 10 minutes sitting or
gardening for more than 2 hours   ain to
e ercises   stretching res_

O   Findings: Visual/Palpable/Test Results

_moderate weakness with sitting Δ L
mo ing from mid thoracic instead of hi s
rib mobility moderately decreased Δ L
breathing restricted-mild Δ_

Modalities: Applications/Locations

_97140   eldenkrais-ribs and thoracic s ine
60 min.   raniosacral-s inal traction and   nwinding_

Response to Treatment (see Δ)

A   Goals: Long-term/Short-term

_all goals ha e been reached within the limits of c rrent
health condition_

Functional Outcomes

_has not regained   rior f nctional stat s since car accident
1-6-01
note acti ities of daily li ing listed abo e_

P   Future Treatment/Frequency

_contin e awareness thro gh mo ement classes once   er month
more often as needed   released from care and referred back to
Dr.   edtree._

Homework/Self-care

_emember to breathe and roll ribs when sitting for long   eriods-
take breaks and do e ercises before stiffness sets in_

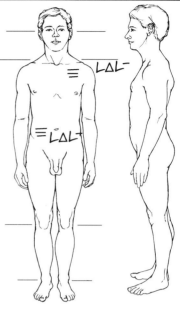

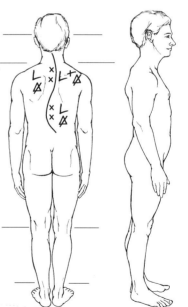

Therapist's Signature   _O L   G_   Date _1-20-05_

Legend: ℮ TP   • TeP   ○ Ⓟ   ⋇ Infl   ≡ HT   ≈ SP

 ✕ Adh   ≷ Numb   ⟳ rot   ╱ elev   ⤛ Short   ↔ Long

101

suggestions for additional care, and any referrals to other caregivers or back to the referring HCP (see Figure 5-7).

Discharge notes include:

◆ Current health status
◆ Summary of treatment
◆ Summary of progress
◆ Reason for ending care
◆ Recommendations for ongoing care
◆ Referrals

Timing

SOAP charting may feel time-consuming at this point. You may be just beginning to chart or you may not have charted this extensively before. Charting may feel burdensome until it becomes habitual and you memorize the standard abbreviations. In time, you can expect to spend considerably less time charting outside each appointment time. Most charting occurs during the session with your clients. Charting in your clients' presence effectively includes them in the healing process. Do this to ensure accuracy and completeness and present an air of professionalism.

Write down subjective and objective information as you gather it from the client. If you are performing hands-on tests or evaluating data at pre-treatment, during the massage, or in post-treatment, take breaks to record information. Recording information as you go will prevent you from forgetting data and will give the client time to rest and integrate your treatment.

After the session is over, review the goals and write new ones. Evaluate the progress and share feedback. Sharing the results of the session aloud immediately after the treatment assists the client in integrating the results, verbalizing his or her needs for the session, and formulating ideas for future solutions. Discuss homework options and write down all assignments. Record the results of the session and status of the goals, write new goals, and work out the treatment plan together before the session ends.

The only thing left to do after the client leaves is to review the subjective and objective data and fill in any details that will assist you in remembering information later. Otherwise, all charting is a part of the session and done with the client present.

Remember, chart extensively every 30 days. Prepare your clients for these comprehensive evaluation sessions by telling them at the initial session what they can expect from the series, including how you work, the importance of gathering information, and how the feedback from the evaluations shapes your treatment plan (and ultimately the results). Impress upon them the importance of the information on your ability to be effective and efficient with your massage, and they will look forward to the information they receive from the assessments you provide.

SUMMARY

SOAP charting is a standard format routinely used by medical, chiropractic, and allied health professionals for documenting health care sessions. SOAP is an acronym that stands for:

◆ Subjective—data provided by the client (symptoms and functional limitations)
◆ Objective—data from the practitioner's perspective (movement tests, palpation findings, visual observations, and treatment and the client's immediate response to the treatment)

- Assessment—functional goals and outcomes based in activities of daily living
- Plan—treatment recommendations and self-care education

Documentation guidelines include:

- Be attentive and practice good listening skills.
- Be clear and concise.
- Measure everything.
- Be specific—avoid vague statements such as improved, better, or less pain.
- Use consistent terminology.
- Chart information pertinent to client's health.
- Be objective.
- Record positive and negative findings.
- Use common medical terms and standard abbreviations.
- Never use correction fluid or eraser to eliminate information.
- Sign or initial each entry with your legal name and credentials.
- Co-sign for students, aides, and apprentices.
- Write legibly.
- Print (or stamp) your name, address, and phone number on each page in the file.

Use a functional outcomes style of reporting information. Set long-term and short-term goals that will clearly demonstrate functional outcomes. Follow SMART criteria for functional goal setting. The SMART acronym stands for:

- Specific—to an activity of daily living
- Measurable—quantify and qualify results to measure progress
- Attainable—success is probable given the client's condition, constitution, and attitude
- Relevant—activity is critical to client's ability to earn a living or care for self, family, or household
- Time-bound—success within a specified time—long-term goals (typically 30 to 60 days) and short-term goals (generally about 1 to 2 weeks)

Describe the symptoms in detail in the Subjective section of the SOAP chart:

- Describe the symptom.
- Note the location.
- Rate the intensity.
- State the duration and frequency.
- Give a detailed description of the onset on the initial SOAP note.

Record functional limitations:

- Identify daily activities the client can no longer do or cannot do without increasing symptoms.
- State the client's previous ability to perform the activities listed.
- State, in measurable terms, the client's current situation regarding the activities.
- Record activities that relieve the client's condition.

Follow these guidelines for documenting objective data:

◆ Document the full range of data.

◆ Measure every finding.

◆ Base measurements on deviations from normal by (1) making bilateral comparison when possible, (2) defining normal for a general population of similar constitution, (3) asking clients to define normal for themselves

◆ Measure the data before and after treatment.

◆ Perform the pre-evaluations and post-evaluations identically.

◆ Chart posture and movement by (1) noting the position of the client, (2) noting the angle of the observation, (3) describing the activity.

◆ Chart palpation by (1) identifying the specific location, (2) rating or describing the touch that triggers the finding, (3) including referred sensations, (4) identifying connections or relationships between findings.

◆ Chart the ROM test by (1) identifying the position of the client, (2) identifying the type of test, (3) naming the joint, (4) naming the action.

◆ Chart the results of the ROM test by (1) rating the amount of movement, (2) rating the pain associated with the movement, (3) rating the quality of the movement.

There are four types of SOAP notes (see Figure 5-8):

◆ Initial—comprehensive, prioritized list of concerns or desired results of the sessions, full-body evaluation, projected goals and treatment plan

◆ Subsequent—focus on treatment, address current concerns and short-term goals and site-specific evaluation

◆ Progress—comprehensive review of concerns, full-body evaluation, evaluate progress and reestablish goals and treatment plan

◆ Discharge—full-body evaluation, summarize health status, summarize progress and functional outcomes, state reason for discharge, make recommendations for ongoing care

Chart throughout the session in the presence of the client to prevent charts from piling up on your desk. Memorize abbreviations and, in time, you will become fast and efficient at SOAP charting.

REFERENCES

1. Kettenbach G. Writing SOAP Notes. 2nd Ed. Philadelphia: FA Davis, 1995.

2. Dolan DW. Insurance Reimbursement and specialty physician referrals. Jacksonville: American Health Press.

3. Rose, MK. The Art of the Chart: Documenting Massage Therapy with CARE Notes. Massage and Body Quarterly April/May, 2003.

4. Bates B. Guide to Physical Examination. 7th Ed. Philadelphia: JB Lippincott, 1999.

5. Magee DJ. Orthopaedic Physical Assessment, 2nd Ed. Philadelphia: WB Saunders, 1992.

6. Adler RH, Giersch P. Whiplash, Spinal Trauma and the Chiropractic Personal Injury Case. 13th Ed. Seattle: Adler◆Giersch, 2000.

7. Travell J, Simons D. Myofascial Pain and Dysfunction: The Trigger Point Massage. Baltimore: Williams & Wilkins, 1983.

FIGURE 5-8 Types of SOAP charts: Comparison of content

	Initial (First visit)	Subsequent	Progress (every 30 Days)	Subsequent	Discharge (last treatment)
S	All Health Concerns **ALL** Symptoms **ALL** Activities of Daily Living	Tx Focus Sx: significant changes only ADLs: significant changes only	Remaining Health Concerns **ALL** Sx **ALL** ADLs	Tx Focus Sx: significant changes only ADLs: significant changes only	Remaining Health Concerns **ALL** Sx **ALL** ADLs
O	**ALL** findings: Visual, palp., mvmt Tx, Δ	findings: significant changes only Tx, Δ	**ALL** findings Tx, Δ	findings: significant changes only Tx, Δ	**ALL** findings Tx, Δ
A	Long-term goals (LTG) Short-term goals (STG)	Functional Outcomes (FOs)	New LTG STG (s)	FOs	any remaining LTG summarize FOs
P	tx plan Homework Selfcare Ex (HW/SC)	HW/SC	New tx plan HW/SC	HW/SC	referral back to HCP long-term HW/SC

The ⟶ means that all data on the previous chart must be addressed in the current chart.

8. Cherkin DC, Eisenberg D, Sherman KJ, Barlow W, Kaptchuk TJ, Street J, Deyo RA. Randomized trial comparing traditional Chinese medical acupuncture, therapeutic massage, and self-care education for chronic low back pain. Arch Intern Med 2001;161:1081.
9. Kendell FP, McCreary EK, Provance PG. Muscles: Testing and Function. 4th Ed. Baltimore: Williams & Wilkins, 1993.
10. Norkin CC, White D. Measurement of Joint Motion: A Guide to Goniometry. Philadelphia: FA Davis, 1995.
11. Chödrön P. Start Where You Are: A Guide to Compassionate Living. Boston: Shambhala, 1994.
12. Weaver R. The Touch Factor Foundation Massage. Montana: Weaver, 1997.

CHAPTER **6**

*E*thics

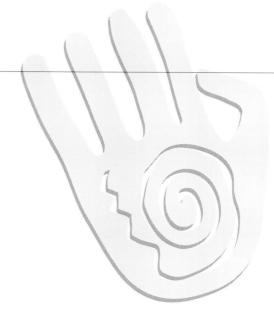

CHAPTER OUTLINE

Annie experienced what anyone would call a miraculous recovery. She had a long history of head and neck trauma, and after a summer of painting the exterior of her house and working long hours at the computer, she ruptured a disk in her neck. The pain was so intense that she could not lift her head high enough to gaze across the horizon, nor could she hold her head up long enough to eat at the dinner table. The numbness and weakness in her right arm was so great that she could not butter her toast or brush her teeth.

Annie's doctor scheduled an MRI. In the meantime, Annie began seeing her Feldenkrais practitioner, John. The first few visits were house calls because riding in a car was excruciating for her—she had to hold her head in her hands and apply traction so the bumps in the road didn't cause more pain than necessary. By the time the results of the MRI came back and the neurosurgeon met with Annie to discuss treatment options, she was pain-free, driving to her own appointments and working part-time. One month from the date of injury, she was working full time and had full mobility in her neck.

John's phone started ringing off the hook. Annie worked in health care, and her peers—amazed by Annie's progress—began referring their clients, friends, and family members to John. But not everyone responded to John's care as Annie had, and several were disappointed when they were not symptom-free after two weeks.

Annie took care of herself in more ways than John knew and in more ways than she told her peers at the clinic. She took naps after every session, limited her activities, and received acupuncture, Tui Na, Polarity, and lymph drainage. She even had a healing session with a Tibetan lama. She began her treatment immediately and aggressively after her injury, getting daily care for the first week—and three times a week for the following three weeks. She had the resources and knowledge to seek treatment that was effective for her, whether or not it was prescribed by her doctor or covered by her insurance. Annie was willing to do whatever it took to get well, she acted quickly, and she never lost sight of her belief that she could heal instantaneously.

John is a brilliant practitioner. He serves all clients equally, to the best of his abilities, given each client's unique situation. The only thing lacking in his sessions has been the conversation about each person's unique healing cycle. Although he made no promises about the results of his treatments, he neglected to address the client's expectations. He, too, had been carried away by his success with Annie. This experience not only increased his skills for working with disk injuries, but also reminded him of the need to communicate clearly with his clients—to hear their expectations and cautiously discuss possible outcomes based on individual circumstances.

Introduction

Webster's defines ethics as the study of standards of conduct and moral judgment. Ethics comes from the Greek word *ethos*, which means the characteristic and distinguishing attitudes, habits, and beliefs of an individual or a group. By definition, massage therapists are students of right and wrong, striving to be moral and just and to respect and uphold the standards of the profession.

With few written guidelines and a great desire to be of service, we learn how to conduct ourselves professionally by taking risks. Life is our classroom; our pursuit of excellence provides the lessons. Obstacles that challenge our sense of fairness and that test our integrity serve to develop our beliefs and shape our character.

As students, we learn by engaging in debates with our peers, questioning our teachers, and consulting our mentors. Through these activities, our visceral and intellectual understanding of right and wrong expands—and our ability to speak honestly, act without fear and greed, and express compassion without prejudice—matures. Eventually, we become role models to others, and our learning expands through interactions with those who seek guidance from us.

As professional massage therapists, we care deeply for our clients and strive to nurture and heal their bodies and souls. In our efforts to be successful, we are influenced by fears, needs, desires, and spiritual longings. Ethical dilemmas are unavoidable. It is critical that we take steps to encourage personal and professional growth and protect those we intend to serve by setting standards for our business practices, evaluating those practices regularly, and discussing ethical beliefs with others. For example:

◆ Define your ethical standards. Write them down. If your professional organization has a code of ethics, frame it and hang it in your office. Read it often.
◆ Create office policies, distribute them to your clients, and stick to them.
◆ Join a supervision group. If you cannot find one, form your own.
◆ Evaluate your business practices and professional relationships monthly.
◆ Invite others to review your business practices annually.
◆ Establish a relationship with a mentor.
◆ Mentor others.

This chapter presents several current ethical dilemmas for massage therapists, specifically in the areas of documentation, treatment practices, and relationships with other health care professionals. It also recommends steps for building and maintaining an ethical practice: a sample code of ethics, a self-evaluation tool for reviewing your business practices and relationships, and an outline for organizing and participating in supervision groups and mentoring. Be a role model for your peers, clients, and other health care providers.

Ethical issues involving emotional and physical relationships between the practitioner and the client—and client confidentiality as it relates to the **Health Insurance Portability and Accountability Act (HIPAA)**—are not discussed in this chapter because of the scope of this subject matter. Many books are dedicated to such topics as boundaries, and HIPAA continues to be debated and clarified. For up-to-date information on client confidentiality specific to HIPAA regulations, contact the U.S. Department of Health and Human Services or visit http://www.aspe.hhs.gov/admnsimp/index.shtml. A resource list of books on ethical issues regarding practitioner-client relationships is provided in Figure 6-1.

Health Insurance Portability and Accountability Act (HIPAA): federal regulation intended to improve the effectiveness and efficiency of the health care system by standardizing the electronic transmission of health information and protecting the security and privacy of health information.

FIGURE 6-1   Resource Books on Ethics

1. Benjamin BE, Sohnen-Moe C. The Ethics of Touch. Tucson, AZ: SMA Inc, 2001.
2. McIntosh N. The Educated Heart: Professional Guidelines for Massage Therapists, Bodyworkers, and Movement Teachers. Memphis, TN: Decatur Bainbridge Press, 1999.
3. Taylor K. The Ethics of Caring: Honoring the Web of Life in our Professional Healing Relationships. 2nd ed. Santa Cruz, CA: Hanford Mead Publishers, 1995.

Current Ethical Dilemmas: Treatment Practices

TREATMENT EXPECTATIONS

At times, clients form expectations of massage therapists based on hearsay. Clients' healing time and abilities vary in many ways, including condition, past history, genetics, emotional complications, and daily physical demands. We may or may not be able to live up to the stories our clients have been told by their friends and family. It is critical to represent our abilities honestly and refrain from committing to specific results or time limits for healing, as we experienced in the opening story about Annie.

Many factors influence healing. As massage therapists, we can only try to find the right combination of modalities, communication techniques, and referrals for each client. Don't take it upon yourself to meet the expectations of everyone who comes to you for help. Instead, talk with each one, find out what her expectations are, tell her what you can honestly predict (which is often nothing more than possibilities), and ask for her help in discovering the best treatment plan for her.

Educate yourself on the state regulations for your profession. Know what claims are legal for your scope of practice. For example, in New York, claims regarding the benefits of massage therapy must be qualified by saying massage therapy "may" reduce inflammation, or "may" improve range of motion (ROM). The only concrete claim permissible is that massage therapy increases circulation.

SCOPE OF PRACTICE

Massage therapy encompasses many modalities and techniques. Much cross-training occurs, often without knowledge of the licensing laws for each profession in each state. A workshop on a massage technique may be taught by an osteopath, with chiropractors, nurses, physical therapists, dentists, and massage therapists as students. Remember that you may be taught techniques that are outside your scope of practice. Receiving training in a technique does not automatically license you to perform it in your practice.

▼

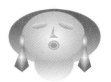

STORY TELLER
Do the Right Thing

Leisha is a massage therapist in Oregon. To escape the cold winter rains, she travels to Hawaii every January for Lomilomi training in the home of an elder Lomi master. Leisha lives there for four weeks every year and adheres to a rigorous schedule of fasting, taking cleansing herbs, and giving and receiving treatments. She learns to harvest the herbs, make cleansing tonics, perform thrust adjustments on the extremities, and apply vigorous manual techniques to increase the circulation. After four years of training, she received the blessing of the elder to provide this healing ritual to others.

Leisha is confident of her skills but knows that Oregon law does not permit her to perform joint manipulations with a thrusting force. Several months go by without temptation. Then, one day, Leisha treats a 40-year-old woman with gnarled, stiff, and painful toes. Leisha knows that the joint manipulations she learned in her Lomi training would benefit this woman, who is prematurely losing mobility in her toes and feet. What should she do?

If the laws that dictate your profession's scope of practice do not adequately represent the skill and training of those licensed, then work to update the laws. Until the laws change, resist the temptation to provide services outside your scope. Create a list of practitioners who can provide those services and refer out when necessary.

TIMELY DOCUMENTATION

Unethical charting practices occur when weeks, months, or years later the chart is filled in because of a request for charts or because payment has been denied and rebilling requires copies of all treatment notes. Charting should be done in a timely fashion. It is difficult to remember a particular session after several other sessions have blurred the details. The best time to chart is during or immediately after the session. We all have days, however, when the charts pile up and we don't get to them until the next morning. It is stressful but possible to recreate the session 24 hours later. However, few of us can record a session accurately weeks, months, or years later.

▼

STORY TELLER
Carbon Dating?

An attorney told a story at a billing seminar of a chiropractor whose notes were carbon dated—a test that establishes the time frame of the record. His client had been injured in a car accident and the attorney for the at-fault-party suspected tampering with the treatment notes and, therefore, ordered the tests. Test results showed that the health care provider had filled in the chart notes 2 to 3 years after the treatments were provided. The client's case was adversely affected.

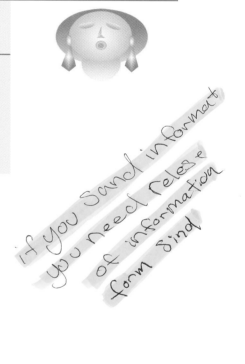

If you Sand informat you need release of information form find

Current Ethical Dilemmas: The Health Care Team
COMMUNICATING WITH HEALTH CARE PROVIDERS

As health care is currently structured, physicians and possibly naturopaths or chiropractors (depending on the insurance policy and the state regulations) are considered primary health care providers (HCPs). It is the primary HCP's responsibility to diagnose the client's problem, orchestrate treatment, and refer to adjunctive therapists, such as massage therapists.

Many of our clients are self-referred, and their HCP may or may not know they are receiving massage therapy. It is imperative to receive permission from clients before communicating with their HCP to avoid any embarassment or conflict between them and their HCP. If you are working under the direction of the **referring HCP** but not under his supervision, good communication is required. In either case, provide the HCP with clear, complete information so that he or she can give the client the best possible treatment.

Occasionally, you may find yourself disagreeing with the HCP about a client's condition or treatment. Do not express this disagreement to the client. Instead, state your views to the HCP—calmly, professionally, tactfully, with all the supporting evidence you can provide. If your input is not considered or if you find that you can't endorse

referring HCP: health care provider who prescribes adjunctive care; often the primary care provider or provider with diagnostic scope authorized to manage the patients' health care

the prescribed treatment, your best choice may be to withdraw from treating the client. However you choose to handle the situation, remember that the HCP is the final authority and that it is unethical for the massage therapist to undermine the relationship between the HCP and the client. If the client approaches you with complaints about the HCP's approach to the treatment plan, support the client in addressing the issues directly with the HCP.

PERMISSION TO CONSULT WITH THE HEALTH CARE TEAM

The health information form contains a request for permission to exchange information with the other members of the client's health care team. In many states, practitioners do not need the client's consent to speak with referring providers, only with adjunctive practitioners. However, if you are bound by HIPAA regulations—whenever you store client information and conduct your transactions electronically—you will need additional documentation to guarentee client confidentiality. Regardless, it is a good idea to inform the client of that and with whom information will be shared.

When providing information to other practitioners, seek written permission, respect the client's confidentiality, and limit those conversations to information pertinent to the client's condition. Omit your personal opinions about the client and any gossip or details that have no bearing on the case. Refrain from discussing any client's cases in public, where others who are not bound by confidentiality can overhear sensitive information.

PAYMENT FOR REFERRALS

We, as massage therapists, are responsible for serving clients to the best of our abilities. Accepting payment for referrals can cloud that ability and compromise our ethics. In all cases, this creates a conflict of interest. In many cases, it is illegal.

rebating: practice of accepting payment for referrals or referring to clinics

The practice of accepting payment for referrals, or referring to clinics or laboratories in which the provider has a financial interest, is known as **rebating**. Severe penalties can be placed on practitioners who violate laws of this nature.

It is appropriate to refer within a health system network or to a preferred provider list. It is not appropriate when the referral is based on the prospect of financial gain.

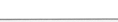

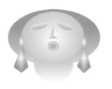

STORY TELLER
Who Is Best for the Client?

Helena's office is centrally located in town. As a result, several HCPs from around the area refer clients to her. One chiropractor on the north end has expanded his office and needs more clients to meet his expenses. He offers Helena $25 for every client she refers to him. Typically, Helena provides a list of chiropractors to clients in need of chiropractic services and highlights those who are located conveniently for the client and who specialize in the area of need. After the chiropractor's offer, Helena begins passing out his card to every client, regardless of which end of town they live and work in or what their special needs for care are.

CODE OF ETHICS

Hang your code of ethics in your office. This code should be one you strive to abide by—one that reflects your beliefs and professional behavior. Many professional organizations have a code of ethics and a disciplinary body to enforce it. Displaying ethical standards instills confidence in clients that their practitioner cares for them, observes a high standard of behavior, and is accountable for his or her actions.

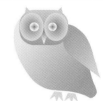

WISE ONE SPEAKS
Code of Ethics

The following is the code of ethics of the American Massage Therapy Association[1]:

This Code of Ethics is a summary statement of the standards by which massage therapists agree to conduct their practice and is a declaration of the general principles of acceptable, ethical, professional behavior.

- Demonstrate commitment to provide the highest quality massage therapy/bodywork to those who seek professional service.
- Acknowledge the inherent worth and individuality of each person by not discriminating or behaving in any prejudicial manner with clients and/or colleagues.
- Demonstrate professional excellence through regular self-assessment of strengths, limitation, and effectiveness by continued education and training.
- Acknowledge the confidential nature of the professional relationship with clients and respect each client's right to privacy.
- Conduct all business and professional activities within their scope of practice, the law of the land, and project a professional image.
- Accept responsibility to do no harm to the physical, mental, and emotional well-being of the self, clients, and associates.
- Refrain from engaging in any sexual conduct or sexual activities involving their clients.

SELF-EVALUATIONS AND PEER EVALUATIONS

Take time to review your business practices and professional relationships. Regular self-evaluations help identify and resolve difficult situations before they become problems.

When you open a new business, establish office policies and a fee schedule, list your services and office hours, and provide copies to all clients. Setting clear boundaries and business parameters helps you treat all clients fairly and equally and provides a comfortable working environment for you and your clients. Review those business guidelines monthly and keep them up to date. Clients become confused and frustrated when policies are distributed to them that no longer apply or are no longer enforced.

As part of your monthly self-evaluation, take 10 minutes to consider the following questions. If your answers highlight a problem situation or call to action, describe the specific situation in writing. Clarify your role in the situation honestly and compassionately. Seek counsel from your peers, if necessary. Identify possible actions and consider the consequences. Determine the timeline for the appropriate action, and follow through.[2]

◆ Did I conduct myself ethically and legally in all my professional affairs?

◆ Did I maintain the confidentiality of my clients?

◆ Did I maintain good boundaries with my clients?

◆ Was I uncomfortable enforcing any office policies? If so, did the situation warrant flexibility or did fear dictate my decision to bend a policy?

◆ What are my strengths and limitations? What action can I take to improve?

◆ What steps have I taken to ensure my well-being?

◆ Are there any issues on which I should seek counsel from my peers?

Annually, review your fee schedule, office policies, and business practices with a peer or a mentor. Review your billing and accounting practices with a professional. Implement changes when appropriate.

CONSULTATION GROUPS

consultation group: a supportive environment in which peers gather to discuss struggles, challenges, and experiences with clients in order to enhance professional development

Consultation groups, also known as peer supervision or co-vision groups, consist of people with a common interest who meet regularly to share ideas, solve problems, and build a community. The common interest can be as broad as massage therapy or as specific as therapists who have clients with AIDS.

Individuals join consultation groups to get support and information, to form professional relationships, and to gain skills. Not only do the people who participate in the consultation groups benefit from the results, but so do their clients, the community, and the profession.

Ethics are difficult to learn out of a book. They must be experienced, experimented with, discussed, and hotly debated. By participating in consultation groups, we can study ethical dilemmas from a variety of perspectives and differing levels of experience, sorting out the possible consequences before our clients can be harmed by our actions. The group members hold one another accountable for telling the truth, express compassion and respect for all involved, and offer advice about confusing issues.[2]

Follow these guidelines for establishing a consultation group in your area:

◆ Define goals for establishing a group.

◆ Identify parameters—how many people, how often will you meet, how long will the meetings last.

◆ Create a list of individuals who have similar goals or needs for a group.

◆ Check the list for individuals you respect and from whom you can learn. It is important to include people who offer diversity to the group, as well as those who share similar opinions.

◆ Select a date for the first meeting. Explain your vision for the group with those on your list and invite them to join you. If you are lacking in numbers, ask those who are interested in being a part of the group to invite others who may also share the same vision.

◆ Get names and phone numbers of those interested, call back to confirm dates and times, and ask for assistance when necessary.

At the first meeting:

◆ Confirm the dates, locations, and times of the meetings. If it is important to the cohesiveness of the group, get a commitment from everyone to attend four consecutive meetings.

◆ Clarify the goals of the group.

◆ Identify the topics of the first few meetings.

◆ Find out whether a mediator, provocateur, or educator is desired for any of the meetings.

◆ Decide whether you want to rotate responsibilities, such as hosting, providing snacks, facilitating the discussion, monitoring the time, and such.

◆ Identify guidelines for group interaction, such as maintaining one another's confidentiality, communicating with respect, and speaking honestly.

◆ Identify guiding principles that suggest ethical behavior without mandating specific rules. For information on identifying guidelines for such occasions, Margaret Wheatly offers guiding principles in her book, *Leadership and the New Science: Take Care of Yourself, Take Care of Each Other, and Take Care of This Place.*[3] Kylea Taylor, in *The Ethics of Caring* defines ethical behavior as reverence for life demonstrated by right relationship and offers Buddha's concepts for right relationship: What I do affects you, what you do affects me, and what I do to you ultimately affects me.[4]

◆ At the end of the meeting, evaluate the outcome. Did you meet your goals? Did you have fun? Make adjustments when necessary to ensure the success of future meetings.

▼

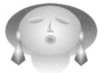

STORY TELLER
A Call to Action

Barb works for a natural foods grocery chain that provides seated massage to customers. There are five stores in her town; each store employs 4 to 5 massage therapists. Barb discovers that providing massage in front of the checkout lines in a grocery store presents problems that she never had to deal with in her private practice, such as maintaining confidentiality. She can tell her coworkers are struggling with the same issues, but she knows it is not appropriate to discuss them at work. She decides to call the practitioners from the stores and try to stir up interest in meeting together and helping one another out with the problems inherent in the work environment.

Barb finds 10 people interested in meeting. She secures a meeting room at the community center and invites one of her teachers from massage school to facilitate the group discussion. She asks a few people to bring snacks and drinks and someone else to make confirmation calls.

Eight of the 23 massage employees attend the meeting. Barb welcomes everyone and introduces the facilitator. The facilitator leads the group in defining the goals for the meeting and identifying topics for discussion. She suggests some guidelines and creates a safe environment for discussion. The group agrees to communicate respectfully and to use a round-robin format to ensure that everyone has the opportunity to speak. The facilitator explains her purpose at the meeting as being one to provide organization and keep the discussion moving in a positive direction, not one of offering her opinion. She begins with a story.

MENTORING

One-on-one consultation lacks the diverse perspectives available in consultation groups, but allows for more spontaneous interactions, more personal attention, and a safe environment for those who find it difficult to speak openly in groups.

Mentors influence and shape us by sharing who they are, not just what they know. The study of ethics is about learning how to live and grow and contribute as a human being, as well as a professional. Select a mentor who is not afraid of sharing his or her mistakes, as well as personal and professional successes. A role model is not a perfect human being, but rather someone who is very much like yourself. Marsha Sinetar, in *The Mentor's Spirit* says, "Show me your mentor and I'll show you yourself."[5]

Select a mentor who:

- Is available weekly by phone
- Is available monthly in person
- Has more professional experience than you
- Is committed to your growth
- Has qualities important to you, such as compassion, wisdom, and ability to confront

SUMMARY

Create an ethical business. Review and revise your business practices regularly. For example:

- Represent your services accurately. Discuss treatment outcomes honestly and realistically.
- Provide services within your scope of practice. Refer out for services that are outside your scope.
- In your charts, do not misrepresent the client's health or the treatment performed.
- Chart client sessions in a timely fashion.
- Discuss disagreements about the treatment plan or client care directly with the HCP, never with the client.
- Support the client in addressing conflicts with other providers directly.
- Request permission from the client to discuss the case with other members of the health care team.
- Limit all conversations with the health care team to information pertinent to the client's condition.
- Be an active student of ethics.
- Develop your ethical beliefs through discussion with peers and mentors.
- Consult your peers and mentors when problems arise in your professional relationships.
- Mentor others.

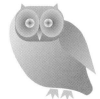

WISE ONE SPEAKS
Discover What Lies Within

I leave you with the following as an inspiration to be in relationship:

It is during interactions with others that we discover what lies within us. That is the gift of our profession—the gift we offer our clients through our listening and the gift we give ourselves through mentoring.

"We usually look outside ourselves for heroes and teachers. It has not occurred to most people that they may already be the role model they seek. The wholeness they are looking for may be trapped within themselves by beliefs, attitudes, and self-doubt. But our wholeness exists in us now. Trapped though it may be, it can be called upon for guidance, direction, and most fundamentally, comfort. It can be remembered. Eventually, we may come to live by it."[6]

1. Code of Ethics. American Massage Therapy Association. Evanston, 2000.
2. Sohnen-Moe C. Business Mastery: A Guide for Creating a Fulfilling and Thriving Business and Keeping It Successful. 3rd Ed. Tucson: Sohnen-Moe Associates, Inc., 1997.
3. Wheatley M. Leadership and the New Science: Learning About Organization From an Orderly Universe. San Francisco: Berrett-Koehler Publishers, Inc., 1994.
4. Taylor K. The Ethics of Caring: Honoring the Web of Life in Our Professional Healing Relationships. 2nd Ed. Santa Cruz: Hanford Mead Publishers, 1995.
5. Sinetar M. The Mentor's Spirit: Life Lessons on Leadership and the Art of Encouragement. Boulder: Sounds True, 1997.
6. Remen RN. Kitchen Table Wisdom: Stories That Heal. New York: Riverhead Books, 1996.

Appendix A
Blank Forms

Blank Forms

* F–female, M–male, non-gender

Description of Forms

1. **Health Information—Wellness Charts** (short version): Healthy clients seeking wellness care fill out the brief health information section at the top of one of these three versions of a Wellness Chart. This information is useful for designing the treatment plan and provides contact information.

Print or stamp your logo, name, and contact information on the top of the page. Photocopy Page 2 of the Wellness Chart (see below) to the back of this form. Clients receiving ongoing care should have individual files. File charts for events by event and date, rather than by client's name.

2. **Health Information** (extended version): Every client with a health concern completes this two-page form annually; more frequently if the client's health condition changes rapidly. This information is useful for designing the treatment plan and provides contact information.

Print or stamp your logo, name, and contact information on the top of each page. Photocopy this form front to back. File completed forms in the client's chart.

3. **Health Report**: The client reports on his or her current condition. This form has multiple uses:

◆ The client completes the form before the session every 30 days as a subjective record of ongoing progress.

◆ The client completes the form before and after the session every 30 days as a subjective record of immediate treatment results and ongoing progress. This requires a two-sided form: Side One is completed before the session; Side Two is completed after the session.

◆ The Health Report can be used as a substitute for a SOAP chart. The client completes Side One before the session and Side Two after the session, as above. The manual therapist records the findings, treatment, and plan in the Comments section.

Print or stamp your logo, name, and contact information on the top of the page. Photocopy front to back, if applicable. This form is available in female, male, and non–gender-specific versions to use at your discretion. Store completed forms in the client's file.

4. **Wellness Charts**: A Wellness note should be written for each massage session performed on a healthy client. There are three types of HxTxC charts provided, any of which can be modified to enhance specific charting needs.

Standard: This is useful for table work—the figures are in a standing position. This form is available in female, male, and non–gender-specific versions to use at your discretion.

Seated: This is useful for on-site sessions—the figures are in a seated position.

Sports: This is useful for sporting events. The intake questions are designed for the treatment needs of athletes before and after competition. Treatments are general and rarely require additional notation.

Print or stamp your logo, name, and contact information on the top of each page. The Standard and Seated Wellness charts include Page 1 (listed above under Health Information) and Page 2, which is suitable for ongoing care. Photocopy both pages together, back-to-back. Page 2 can also be photocopied back-to-back, because the intake form only needs to be completed annually or biannually. The Wellness Chart—Sports only has one page and can be photocopied back-to-back.

Clients receiving ongoing care should have individual files. File charts for events by event and date, rather than by client's name.

5. **SOAP Charts**: A SOAP note should be written for each curative treatment session. There are two styles of SOAP forms used for recording the various types of SOAP notes:

Long version—Use the full page SOAP chart for Initial notes, Progress notes, Discharge notes, or any time additional space is required.

Short version—Use the half page SOAP chart for subsequent notes or health conditions that do not require extensive space for recording information.

Print or stamp your logo, name, and contact information on the top of each page. Photocopy the long version as Page 1 and the short version as Page 2. Also, photocopy the short version back to back. This chart is available in female, male, and non–gender-specific versions to use at your discretion. File completed forms in the client's chart.

6. **Range of Motion**: Use this for ease in charting range of motion tests. Space is provided for pre-treatment and post-treatment assessment for up to three joint assessments or you may use one form for up to three sessions, if you are only assessing the motion of one joint. If you photocopy back-to-back, one piece of paper can be used for up to six treatment sessions, or, photocopy onto the back of a Health Report to be used every 30 days for noting ongoing progress.

Print or stamp your logo, name, and contact information on the top of the page. Store completed forms in the client's file.

Massage Therapist _____   **WELLNESS CHART-F**

Name _____ ID#/DOB _____ Date _____

Phone _____ Address _____

1. What are your goals for health, and how may I assist you in achieving your goals? _____

   _____

2. List typical daily activities—work, exercise, home. _____

   _____

3. Are you currently experiencing any of the following? If yes, please explain.

   pain, tenderness   ☐ No ☐ Yes: _____   stiffness ☐ No ☐ Yes: _____
   numbness or tingling   ☐ No ☐ Yes: _____   swelling   ☐ No ☐ Yes: _____
   allergies   ☐ No ☐ Yes: _____

4. List all illnesses, injuries, and health concerns you have now or have had in the past 3 years.
   (Examples: arthritis, diabetes, car crash, pregnancy) _____

   _____

5. List medications and pain relievers taken this week. _____

6. I have provided all my known medical information. I acknowledge that massage therapy is
   not a substitute for medical diagnosis and treatment. I give my consent to receive treatment.

   Signature _____ Date _____

   Tx: _____

   _____

   C: _____

   _____

Legend:

℮ TP	● TeP	○ ⓟ	✳ Infl	☰ HT	≈ SP	initials _____
✕ Adh	≷ Numb	↻ rot	╱ elev	⤚ Short	⟷ Long	

124   Copyright © 2005 Lippincott Williams & Wilkins

Massage Therapist _____ **WELLNESS CHART-M**

Name _____ ID#/DOB _____ Date _____

Phone _____ Address _____

1. What are your goals for health, and how may I assist you in achieving your goals? _____
   _____

2. List typical daily activities—work, exercise, home. _____
   _____

3. Are you currently experiencing any of the following? If yes, please explain.

   pain, tenderness   ☐ No ☐ Yes: _____   stiffness ☐ No ☐ Yes: _____
   numbness or tingling   ☐ No ☐ Yes: _____   swelling ☐ No ☐ Yes: _____
   allergies   ☐ No ☐ Yes: _____

4. List all illnesses, injuries, and health concerns you have now or have had in the past 3 years.
   (Examples: arthritis, diabetes, car crash, pregnancy) _____
   _____

5. List medications and pain relievers taken this week. _____

6. I have provided all my known medical information. I acknowledge that massage therapy is
   not a substitute for medical diagnosis and treatment. I give my consent to receive treatment.

   Signature _____ Date _____

   Tx: _____
   _____

   C: _____
   _____

Legend:

℮ TP	• TeP	○ Ⓟ	⚹ Infl	≡ HT	≈ SP initials _____
✕ Adh	≋ Numb	↻ rot	╱ elev	⊱⊰ Short	↔ Long

125

Massage Therapist _____ **WELLNESS CHART**

Name _____ ID#/DOB _____ Date _____

Phone _____ Address _____

1. What are your goals for health, and how may I assist you in achieving your goals? _____
   _____

2. List typical daily activities—work, exercise, home. _____
   _____

3. Are you currently experiencing any of the following? If yes, please explain.

pain, tenderness	☐ No ☐ Yes: _____	stiffness	☐ No ☐ Yes: _____
numbness or tingling	☐ No ☐ Yes: _____	swelling	☐ No ☐ Yes: _____
allergies	☐ No ☐ Yes: _____		

4. List all illnesses, injuries, and health concerns you have now or have had in the past 3 years.
   (Examples: arthritis, diabetes, car crash, pregnancy) _____
   _____

5. List medications and pain relievers taken this week. _____

6. I have provided all my known medical information. I acknowledge that massage therapy is
   not a substitute for medical diagnosis and treatment. I give my consent to receive treatment.

   Signature _____ Date _____

   Tx: _____
   _____

   C: _____

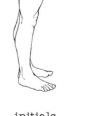

Legend:

℮ TP   ● TeP   ○ Ⓟ   ✳ Infl   ☰ HT   ≈ SP   initials _____

✕ Adh   ≋ Numb   ↺ rot   ╱ elev   ↣ Short   ↔ Long

126

Massage Therapist

WELLNESS CHART—SEATED

Name _____ ID#/DOB _____ Date _____

Phone _____ Address _____

1. What are your goals for health, and how may I assist you in achieving your goals? _____
   _____

2. List typical daily activities—work, exercise, home. _____
   _____

3. Are you currently experiencing any of the following? If yes, please explain.

pain, tenderness	☐ No ☐ Yes: _____	stiffness ☐ No ☐ Yes: _____
numbness or tingling	☐ No ☐ Yes: _____	swelling ☐ No ☐ Yes: _____
allergies	☐ No ☐ Yes: _____	

4. List all illnesses, injuries, and health concerns you have now or have had in the past 3 years.
   (Examples: arthritis, diabetes, car crash, pregnancy) _____
   _____

5. List medications and pain relievers taken this week. _____

6. I have provided all my known medical information. I acknowledge that massage therapy is
   not a substitute for medical diagnosis and treatment. I give my consent to receive treatment.

   Signature _____ Date _____

   Tx: _____
   _____

   C: _____
   _____

initials _____

Legend:

ℰ TP	• TeP	○ Ⓟ	✳ Infl	≡ HT	≈ SP
✕ Adh	≋ Numb	↻ rot	╱ elev	⤞ Short	⟷ Long

WELLNESS CHART—SPORTS

Massage Therapist _____ Date _____

Event _____ Location _____

Ask each athlete the following: (Note individual responses below—concerns only.)

1. Are you currently experiencing any of the following?
   - pain, tenderness, stiffness
   - numbness, tingling
   - cold, clammy skin
   - swelling
   - dizziness
   - shaking

2. How soon do you compete? / When did you finish competing?

3. Have you warmed up? / Cooled down?

4. Have you consumed water since the event?

Athlete's Name _____ Athlete's initials: _____

Hx: (note concerns) _____

Tx: (check all that apply) _____ Pre-event _____ Post-event _____ Refer-first aid/med

C: _____ Initials: _____

Athlete's Name _____ Athlete's initials: _____

Hx: (note concerns) _____

Tx: (check all that apply) _____ Pre-event _____ Post-event _____ Refer-first aid/med

C: _____ Initials: _____

Athlete's Name _____ Athlete's initials: _____

Hx: (note concerns) _____

Tx: (check all that apply) _____ Pre-event _____ Post-event _____ Refer-first aid/med

C: _____ Initials: _____

Athlete's Name _____ Athlete's initials: _____

Hx: (note concerns) _____

Tx: (check all that apply) _____ Pre-event _____ Post-event _____ Refer-first aid/med

C: _____ Initials: _____

Athlete's Name _____ Athlete's initials: _____

Hx: (note concerns) _____

Tx: (check all that apply) _____ Pre-event _____ Post-event _____ Refer-first aid/med

C: _____ Initials: _____

Athlete's Name _____ Athlete's initials: _____

Hx: (note concerns) _____

Tx: (check all that apply) _____ Pre-event _____ Post-event _____ Refer-first aid/med

C: _____ Initials: _____

Massage Therapist _____ **HEALTH INFORMATION**

Client Name _____ Date _____

Date of Injury _____ ID#/DOB _____

A. Client Information

Address _____

City _____ State ____ Zip _____

Phone: Home _____

   Work _____ Cell _____

Employer _____

Work Address _____

Occupation _____

Emergency Contact _____

Phone: Home _____

   Work _____ Cell _____

Primary Health Care Provider

Name _____

Address _____

City/State/Zip _____

Phone: _____ Fax _____

I give my massage therapist permission to consult with my health care providers regarding my health and treatment.

Comments _____

Initials _____ Date _____

B. Current Health Information

List Health Concerns Check all that apply

Primary _____
- [ ] mild [ ] moderate [ ] disabling
- [ ] constant [ ] intermittant
- [ ] symptoms ↑ w/activity [ ] ↓ w/activity
- [ ] getting worse [ ] getting better [ ] no change

treatment received _____

Secondary _____
- [ ] mild [ ] moderate [ ] disabling
- [ ] constant [ ] intermittant
- [ ] symptoms ↑ w/activity [ ] ↓ w/activity
- [ ] getting worse [ ] getting better [ ] no change

treatment received _____

Additional _____
- [ ] mild [ ] moderate [ ] disabling
- [ ] constant [ ] intermittant
- [ ] symptoms ↑ w/activity [ ] ↓ w/activity
- [ ] getting worse [ ] getting better [ ] no change

treatment received _____

List Daily Activities Limited by Condition

Work _____

_____

Home/Family _____

_____

Sleep/Self-care _____

Social/Recreational _____

List Self-Care Routines

How do you reduce stress? _____

_____

Pain? _____

_____

List current medications (include pain relievers and herbal remedies) _____

_____

_____

_____

Have you ever received massage therapy before? _____ Frequency? _____

What are your goals for receiving massage therapy? _____

_____

_____

C. Health History

List and Explain. Include dates and treatment received.

Surgeries _____

_____

_____

_____

Injuries _____

_____

_____

Major Illnesses _____

_____

_____

Check All Current and Previous Conditions Please Explain

General

current	past		comments
☐	☐	headaches	_____
☐	☐	pain	_____
☐	☐	sleep disturbances	
			_____
☐	☐	fatigue	_____
☐	☐	infections	_____
☐	☐	fever	_____
☐	☐	sinus	_____
☐	☐	other	_____

Skin Conditions

current	past		comments
☐	☐	rashes	_____
☐	☐	athlete's foot, warts	_____
☐	☐	other	_____

Muscles and Joints

current	past		comments
☐	☐	rheumatoid arthritis	
			_____
☐	☐	osteoarthritis	_____
			_____
☐	☐	osteoporosis	_____
☐	☐	scoliosis	_____
☐	☐	broken bones	_____
☐	☐	spinal problems	_____
			_____
☐	☐	disk problems	_____
☐	☐	lupus	_____
☐	☐	TMJ, jaw pain	_____
☐	☐	spasms, cramps	
			_____
☐	☐	sprains, strains	
☐	☐	tendonitis, bursitis	
			_____
☐	☐	stiff or painful joints	_____
☐	☐	weak or sore muscles	
			_____
☐	☐	neck, shoulder, arm pain	
☐	☐	low back, hip, leg pain	
			_____
☐	☐	other	_____

Nervous System

current	past		comments
☐	☐	head injuries, concussions	
			_____
☐	☐	dizziness, ringing in ears	
☐	☐	loss of memory, confusion	
			_____
☐	☐	numbness, tingling	
☐	☐	sciatica, shooting pain	
			_____
☐	☐	chronic pain	_____
☐	☐	depression	_____
☐	☐	other	_____

Respiratory, Cardiovascular

current	past		comments
☐	☐	heart disease	_____
			_____
☐	☐	blood clots	_____
☐	☐	stroke	_____
☐	☐	lymphadema	_____
☐	☐	high, low blood pressure	
☐	☐	irregular heart beat	
			_____
☐	☐	poor circulation	_____
☐	☐	swollen ankles	_____
☐	☐	varicose veins	_____
☐	☐	chest pain, shortness of breath	_____
☐	☐	asthma	_____

Allergies

current	past		comments
☐	☐	scents, oils, lotions	_____
☐	☐	detergents	_____
☐	☐	other	_____

Digestive/Elimination System

current	past		comments
☐	☐	bowel problems	_____
			_____
☐	☐	gas, bloating	_____
☐	☐	bladder/kidney/prostrate	
☐	☐	abdominal pain	_____
☐	☐	other	_____

Endocrine System

current	past		comments
☐	☐	thyroid	_____
☐	☐	diabetes	_____

Reproductive System

current	past		comments
☐	☐	pregnancy	_____
			_____
☐	☐	painful, emotional menses	
			_____
☐	☐	fibrotic cysts	_____

Cancer/Tumors

current	past		comments
☐	☐	benign	_____
☐	☐	malignant	_____

Habits

current	past		comments
☐	☐	tobacco	_____
☐	☐	alcohol	_____
☐	☐	drugs	_____
☐	☐	coffee, soda	_____

Contract for Care

I promise to participate fully as a member of my health care team. I will make sound choices regarding my treatment plan based on the information provided by my massage therapist and other members of my health care team, and my experience of those suggestions. I agree to participate in the self care program we select. I promise to inform my practitioner any time I feel my well-being is threatened or compromised. I expect my massage therapist to provide safe and effective treatment.

Consent for Care

It is my choice to receive massage therapy, and I give my consent to receive treatment. I have reported all health conditions that I am aware of and will inform my practitioner of any changes in my health.

Signature _____ Date _____

Massage Therapist _____   **HEALTH REPORT-F**

Client Name _____ Date _____

Date of Injury _____ ID#/DOB _____

A. Draw today's symptoms on the figures.

1. Identify CURRENT symptomatic areas in your body by marking letters on the figures below. Use the letters provided in the key to identify the symptoms you are feeling today.
2. Circle the area around each letter, representing the size and shape of each symptom location.

Key

P = pain or tenderness
S = joint or muscle stiffness
N = numbness or tingling

B. Identify the intensity of your symptoms.

1. Pain Scale: Mark a line on the scale to show the amount of pain you are experiencing today.

   No Pain ├──┤ Unbearable Pain

2. Activities Scale: Mark a line on the scale to show the limitations you are experiencing today in your daily activities.

   Can Do Anything I Want ├──────────────────────────────┤ Cannot Do Anything

C. Comments

_____
_____
_____
_____

Signature _____ Date _____

131

Massage Therapist   **HEALTH REPORT-M**

Client Name _____ Date _____

Date of Injury _____ ID#/DOB

A. Draw today's symptoms on the figures.

1. Identify CURRENT symptomatic areas in your body by marking letters on the figures below. Use the letters provided in the key to identify the symptoms you are feeling today.
2. Circle the area around each letter, representing the size and shape of each symptom location.

Key
P = pain or tenderness
S = joint or muscle stiffness
N = numbness or tingling

B. Identify the intensity of your symptoms.

1. Pain Scale: Mark a line on the scale to show the amount of pain you are experiencing today.

No Pain |———————————————————————————————| Unbearable Pain

2. Activities Scale: Mark a line on the scale to show the limitations you are experiencing today in your daily activities.

Can Do Anything I Want |———————————————————————————| Cannot Do Anything

C. Comments

_____
_____
_____
_____

Signature _____ Date _____

Massage Therapist _____ **HEALTH REPORT**

Client Name _____ Date _____

Date of Injury _____ ID#/DOB _____

A. Draw today's symptoms on the figures.

1. Identify CURRENT symptomatic areas in your body by marking letters on the figures below. Use the letters provided in the key to identify the symptoms you are feeling today.
2. Circle the area around each letter, representing the size and shape of each symptom location.

Key
P = pain or tenderness
S = joint or muscle stiffness
N = numbness or tingling

B. Identify the intensity of your symptoms.

1. Pain Scale: Mark a line on the scale to show the amount of pain you are experiencing today.

   No Pain ├──────────────────────────────────┤ Unbearable Pain

2. Activities Scale: Mark a line on the scale to show the limitations you are experiencing today in your daily activities.

   Can Do Anything I Want ├──────────────────────────────────┤ Cannot Do Anything

C. Comments

_____
_____
_____
_____

Signature _____ Date _____

Massage Therapist _____   **WELLNESS CHART—F**

Name _____ ID#/DOB _____ Meds _____

Tx: _____

C: _____

_____

date _____ initials _____

Tx: _____

C: _____

_____

date _____ initials _____

Tx: _____

C: _____

_____

date _____ initials _____

Tx: _____

C: _____

_____

date _____ initials _____

Legend:

℮ TP	• TeP	○ Ⓟ	✳ Infl	≡ HT	≈ SP
✕ Adh	≋ Numb	⟲ rot	╱ elev	⊱ Short	⟷ Long

Massage Therapist _____ **WELLNESS CHART—M**

Name _____ ID#/DOB _____ Meds _____

Tx: _____   Tx: _____

_____

C: _____   C: _____

_____

date _____ initials _____   date _____ initials _____

Tx: _____   Tx: _____

_____

C: _____   C: _____

_____

date _____ initials _____   date _____ initials _____

Legend: ℮ TP   • TeP   ○ Ⓟ   ⁎ Infl   ≡ HT   ≈ SP

          ✕ Adh   ≷ Numb   ↻ rot   ╱ elev   >—< Short   ↔ Long

Massage Therapist _____   **WELLNESS CHART**

Name _____ ID#/DOB _____ Meds _____

Tx: _____   Tx: _____
    _____   _____
C: _____   C: _____
   _____   _____

date _____ initials _____   date _____ initials _____

Tx: _____   Tx: _____
    _____   _____
C: _____   C: _____
   _____   _____

date _____ initials _____   date _____ initials _____

Legend: ℰ TP   • TeP   ○ ℗   ⋇ Infl   ≡ HT   ≈ SP
              ✕ Adh   ≋ Numb   ⟲ rot   ╱ elev   ⊢ Short   ↔ Long

136   Copyright © 2005 Lippincott Williams & Wilkins

WELLNESS CHART—SEATED

Name _____ ID#/DOB _____ Meds _____

Tx: _____   Tx: _____

_____   _____

C: _____   C: _____

_____   _____

date _____ initials _____   date _____ initials _____

Tx: _____   Tx: _____

C: _____   C: _____

_____   _____

date _____ initials _____   date _____ initials _____

Legend:

℮ TP	● TeP	○ Ⓟ	✳ Infl	≡ HT	≈ SP
✕ Adh	≳ Numb	⌒ rot	╱ elev	⪤ Short	↔ Long

137

Massage Therapist _____ **SOAP CHART-F**

Client Name _____ Date _____

Date of Injury _____ ID#/DOB _____ Meds _____

S Focus/Health Concerns: Prioritize

Symptoms: Location/Intensity/Frequency/Duration/Onset

Activities of Daily Living: Aggravating/Relieving

O Findings: Visual/Palpable/Test Results

Techniques/Modalities: Locations/Duration

Response to Treatment (see Δ)

A Goals: Long-term/Short-term

Functional Outcomes

P Future Treatment/Frequency

Homework/Self-care

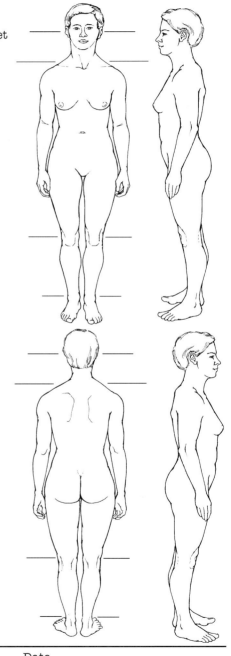

Therapist's Signature _____ Date _____

Legend: ℮ TP   • TeP   ○ Ⓟ   ⋇ Infl   ≡ HT   ≈ SP

✕ Adh   ≳ Numb   ◠ rot   ╱ elev   ⊶ Short   ↔ Long

Massage Therapist _____

SOAP CHART-M

Client Name _____ Date _____

Date of Injury _____ ID#/DOB _____ Meds _____

S Focus/Health Concerns: Prioritize

Symptoms: Location/Intensity/Frequency/Duration/Onset

Activities of Daily Living: Aggravating/Relieving

O Findings: Visual/Palpable/Test Results

Techniques/Modalities: Locations/Duration

Response to Treatment (see Δ)

A Goals: Long-term/Short-term

Functional Outcomes

P Future Treatment/Frequency

Homework/Self-care

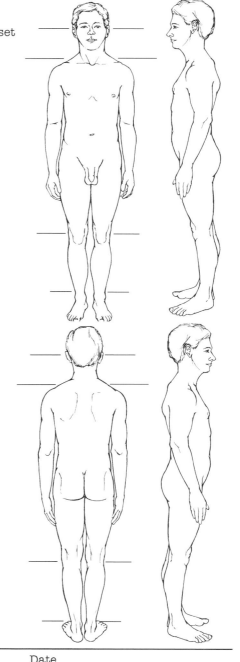

Therapist's Signature _____ Date _____

Legend:

℮ TP	• TeP	○ Ⓟ	✳ Infl	☰ HT	≈ SP
✕ Adh	≋ Numb	↻ rot	╱ elev	⊶ Short	↔ Long

139

Massage Therapist _____ **SOAP CHART**

Client Name _____ Date _____

Date of Injury _____ ID#/DOB _____ Meds _____

S Focus/Health Concerns: Prioritize

Symptoms: Location/Intensity/Frequency/Duration/Onset

Activities of Daily Living: Aggravating/Relieving

O Findings: Visual/Palpable/Test Results

Techniques/Modalities: Locations/Duration

Response to Treatment (see Δ)

A Goals: Long-term/Short-term

Functional Outcomes

P Future Treatment/Frequency

Homework/Self-care

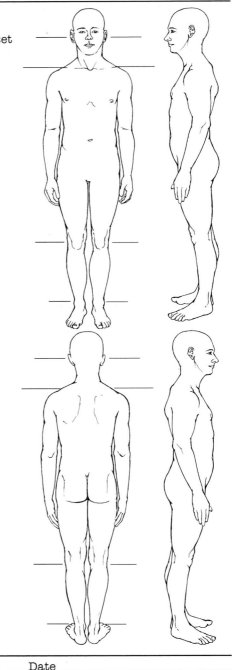

Therapist's Signature _____ Date _____

Legend: ℮ TP   • TeP   ○ ℗   ⃟ Infl   ≡ HT   ≈ SP
                ✕ Adh   ≷ Numb   ↻ rot   ╱ elev   ⊶ Short   ↔ Long

140   Copyright © 2005 Lippincott Williams & Wilkins

Massage Therapist _____   **SOAP CHART-F**

Client Name _____ Date _____

Date of Injury _____ ID#/DOB _____ Meds _____

S

O

A

P

_____

Therapist's Signature _____ Date _____

S

O

A

P

_____

Therapist's Signature _____ Date _____

Legend:

ℭ TP	● TeP	○ Ⓟ	✳ Infl	≡ HT	≈ SP
✕ Adh	≋ Numb	⟲ rot	╱ elev	⊶ Short	⟷ Long

Massage Therapist _____

Client Name _____ Date _____

Date of Injury _____ ID#/DOB _____ Meds _____

S

O

A

P

Therapist's Signature _____ Date _____

S

O

A

P

Therapist's Signature _____ Date _____

Legend: © TP   • TeP   ◯ Ⓟ   ✱ Infl   ≡ HT   ≈ SP

         ✕ Adh   ≳ Numb   ⚆ rot   / elev   ⋜ Short   ⟷ Long

142   Copyright © 2005 Lippincott Williams & Wilkins

Massage Therapist _____ **SOAP CHART**

Client Name _____ Date _____

Date of Injury _____ ID#/DOB _____ Meds _____

S

O

A

P

Therapist's Signature _____ Date _____

S

O

A

P

Therapist's Signature _____ Date _____

Legend: ℮ TP   ● TeP   ○ Ⓟ   ✳ Infl   ≡ HT   ≈ SP

✕ Adh   ≳ Numb   ⬯ rot   ╱ elev   ⊢ Short   ⟷ Long

RANGE OF MOTION

Client Name _____ Date _____

Date of Injury _____ ID#/DOB _____

PRE-TEST 1 Initials _____ Date _____

Position of patient: prone, sidelying, sitting, standing, supine, other: _____

Type of test: active, active assisted, passive, resistive, other: _____

Joint: C-spine, T-spine, L-spine, hip, knee, ankle, shoulder, elbow, wrist, other: _____

Action	Quantify ↓ or ↑		Rate Pain		Rate Quality	
	ⓇR	ⓁL	ⓇR	ⓁL	ⓇR	ⓁL

POST-TEST 1 Initials _____ Date _____

Position of patient: prone, sidelying, sitting, standing, supine, other: _____

Type of test: active, active assisted, passive, resistive, other: _____

Joint: C-spine, T-spine, L-spine, hip, knee, ankle, shoulder, elbow, wrist, other: _____

Action	Quantify ↓ or ↑		Rate Pain		Rate Quality	
	Ⓡ	Ⓛ	Ⓡ	Ⓛ	Ⓡ	Ⓛ

PRE-TEST 2 Initials _____ Date _____

Position of patient: prone, sidelying, sitting, standing, supine, other: _____

Type of test: active, active assisted, passive, resistive, other: _____

Joint: C-spine, T-spine, L-spine, hip, knee, ankle, shoulder, elbow, wrist, other: _____

Action	Quantify ↓ or ↑		Rate Pain		Rate Quality	
	Ⓡ	Ⓛ	Ⓡ	Ⓛ	Ⓡ	Ⓛ

POST-TEST 2 Initials _____ Date _____

Position of patient: prone, sidelying, sitting, standing, supine, other: _____

Type of test: active, active assisted, passive, resistive, other: _____

Joint: C-spine, T-spine, L-spine, hip, knee, ankle, shoulder, elbow, wrist, other: _____

Action	Quantify ↓ or ↑		Rate Pain		Rate Quality	
	Ⓡ	Ⓛ	Ⓡ	Ⓛ	Ⓡ	Ⓛ

PRE-TEST 3 Initials _____ Date _____

Position of patient: prone, sidelying, sitting, standing, supine, other: _____

Type of test: active, active assisted, passive, resistive, other: _____

Joint: C-spine, T-spine, L-spine, hip, knee, ankle, shoulder, elbow, wrist, other: _____

Action	Quantify ↓ or ↑		Rate Pain		Rate Quality	
	Ⓡ	Ⓛ	Ⓡ	Ⓛ	Ⓡ	Ⓛ

POST-TEST 3 Initials _____ Date _____

Position of patient: prone, sidelying, sitting, standing, supine, other: _____

Type of test: active, active assisted, passive, resistive, other: _____

Joint: C-spine, T-spine, L-spine, hip, knee, ankle, shoulder, elbow, wrist, other: _____

Action	Quantify ↓ or ↑		Rate Pain		Rate Quality	
	Ⓡ	Ⓛ	Ⓡ	Ⓛ	Ⓡ	Ⓛ

Directions for charting Range of Motion Results: For each test, fill in the form blanks as follows:
ACTION—Identify the action tested: abd, add, DF, ever, ext, ext rot, flex, int rot, inv, lat flex, PF, pro, SB, and Sup
QUANTIFY—Quantify the available range of motion: ↓ (hypomobility), ↑ (hypermobility); L, M, S; 0–10; N, G, F, P (Normal, Good, Fair, Poor).
PAIN—Identify if Pain is present with movement: If present, rate pain. If absent: Ø.
QUALITY—Identify and Rate the quality of movement: sm, seg, Sp, rig (smooth, segmented, spastic, rigid)

Appendix B
Case Studies

Documentation for Wellness Massage—Seated

Case Study: Tham Maad, a 24-year-old male, is a computer programmer who works long hours, and when he finally goes home, he spends time e-mailing his family overseas and playing computer games. Lately, he has been experiencing mild stiffness in his right shoulder and mild numbness and tingling in his right arm and hand. His symptoms increase to moderate late in the day, requiring him to take frequent breaks from the computer. Sometimes, his hand is numb when we wakes up in the morning, but the feeling comes right back with use. The company he works for has recently hired a massage company to provide seated massage in the break room twice a week. The massages are subsidized by the company, and Tham is ready to take advantage of the deal—anything to be able to work more. His first massage is a 30-minute session, and he reschedules for weekly sessions.

Flow Charts: This flow chart demonstrates the forms that are recommended for use with clients seeking wellness massage in an on-site environment: who completes the form, how often the form is used, and any additional comments for using the form.

Wellness Care	Who	Frequency	Comments
INTAKE FORMS			
Fees and Policies	Client	Initial visit	Update as needed
Health Info—short version	Client	Initial visit	Update annually
Health Info—long version	—		
PROGRESS SUMMARIES			
Health Report	Client	Initial visit	Update every 6 to 8 tx
Progress Report	—		
TREATMENT NOTES			
Wellness Chart	MT	Each visit	Record treatment; findings
Initial SOAP—long version	—		
Subsequent SOAP—short version	—		
Progress SOAP—long version	—		
Discharge SOAP—long version	—		
Range of Motion	—		

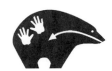

Sarah Benjamin
123 Sun Moon and Stars Drive
Capitol Hill, WA   98119
Tel   206 555 4446

FEES AND POLICIES

A. Fee schedule

- Chair Massage $10/$20   15 minutes
- Chair Massage $30/$40   30 mintues

Microtech pays for the first $10 of each massage for up to four massages per calandar month. The first price listed is the subsidized price, the second price listed is the fee for all massages received after the limit has been met.

B. Payment Policies

Please make all co-payments at the time of service. Microtech will be billed for the remainder at the end of each month.

C. Office Policies

Cancellations

Cancellations must be made by noon the previous business day, or the co-payment will be collected. This charge will be waived if a replacement can be found for your appointment time. Microtech will not be billed for your no-shows or late cancellations.

Privacy

Please respect the privacy of the other people receiving massages at the same time as you. There will often be two massages going on at the same time. Please speak in whispers and do not repeat anything you may overhear outside of the massage room.

Comfort and Dress

Some people prefer to remove their contact lenses for the massage. Be prepared to do so, so you can fully relax. If you think you would be more comfortable, bring a cotton T-shirt to change into for your massage. Thick sweaters and jackets and tight belts should be removed. If you wear make-up, bring your kit with you to work, as it may smear during your massage. You may prefer to use make-up sparingly on the day of your massage, or wash it off prior to your session.

Client Agreement

I have read the policies stated above and agree to abide by them.

Signature _Tham Maad_____ Date _12-12-04_____

WELLNESS CHART—SEATED

Name __Tham Maad__ ID#/DOB __12-19-80__ Date __12-12-04__

Phone __ext 134__ Address __Microtech N. campus 2nd floor__

1. What are your goals for health, and how may I assist you in achieving your goals? _____
   __work without numbness, relax__

2. List typical daily activities—work, exercise, home. __computer, reading, skateboarding__
   _____

3. Are you currently experiencing any of the following? If yes, please explain.

   pain, tenderness   ☒ No   ☐ Yes: _____   stiffness   ☐ No   ☒ Yes: __R SH__
   numbness or tingling   ☐ No   ☒ Yes: __R hand__   swelling   ☒ No   ☐ Yes: _____
   allergies   ☒ No   ☐ Yes: _____

4. List all illnesses, injuries, and health concerns you have now or have had in the past 3 years.
   (Examples: arthritis, diabetes, car crash, pregnancy) __MVC Aug. 1993__
   _____

5. List medications and pain relievers taken this week. __none__

6. I have provided all my known medical information. I acknowledge that massage therapy is
   not a substitute for medical diagnosis and treatment. I give my consent to receive treatment.

   Signature __Tham Maad__ Date __12-12-04__

   Tx: __30 min. SW (M) – Focus on (R) SH, arm, hand, BL neck, chest, back, light pressure__

   C: __tingling in (R) hand radiates from (R) elbow, intermittant, worse in AM and late afternoon__

initials __SB, UMT__

Legend: ℮ TP   • TeP   ○ (P)   ✳ Infl   ≡ HT   ≈ SP
     ✕ Adh   ≋ Numb   ⟲ rot   ∕ elev   ⊢ Short   ↔ Long

Sarah Benjamin
123 Sun Moon and Stars Drive
Capitol Hill, WA   98119
TEL   206 555 4446

HEALTH REPORT

Client Name _Tham Maad_   Date _12-12-04_

Date of Injury _N/A_   ID#/DOB _12-19-80_

A. Draw today's symptoms on the figures.

1. Identify CURRENT symptomatic areas in your body by marking letters on the figures below. Use the letters provided in the key to identify the symptoms you are feeling today.
2. Circle the area around each letter, representing the size and shape of each symptom location.

Key
P = pain or tenderness
S = joint or muscle stiffness
N = numbness or tingling

B. Identify the intensity of your symptoms.

1. Pain Scale: Mark a line on the scale to show the amount of pain you are experiencing today.

   No Pain |————————————————————————————| Unbearable Pain

2. Activities Scale: Mark a line on the scale to show the limitations you are experiencing today in your daily activities.

   Can Do Anything I Want |———|————————————————| Cannot Do Anything

C. Comments

Sometimes, after a long day at work, the numbness makes me take several breaks from the computer—today is one of those days.

Signature _Tham Maad_   Date _12-12-04_

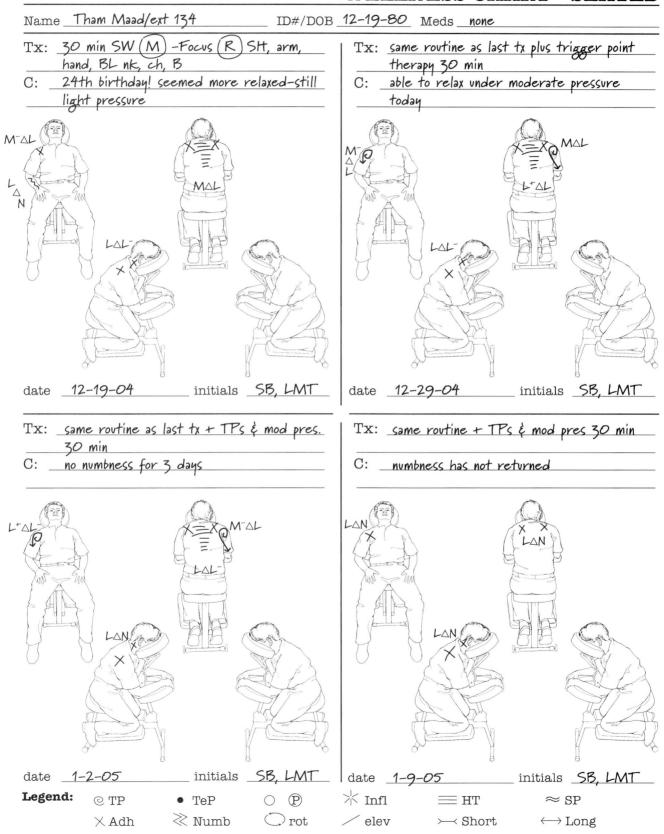

Sarah Benjamin
123 Sun Moon and Stars Drive
Capitol Hill, WA   98119
Tel   206 555 4446

WELLNESS CHART—SEATED

Name _Tham Maad/ext 134_   ID#/DOB _12-19-80_   Meds _none_

Tx: 30 min SW (M) -Focus (R) SH, arm,
       hand, BL nk, ch, B
C: 24th birthday! seemed more relaxed-still
       light pressure

date _12-19-04_   initials SB, LMT

Tx: same routine as last tx plus trigger point
       therapy 30 min
C: able to relax under moderate pressure
       today

date _12-29-04_   initials SB, LMT

Tx: same routine as last tx + TPs & mod pres.
       30 min
C: no numbness for 3 days

date _1-2-05_   initials SB, LMT

Tx: same routine + TPs & mod pres 30 min
C: numbness has not returned

date _1-9-05_   initials SB, LMT

Legend:
    ℮ TP   • TeP   ○ Ⓟ   ✳ Infl   ≡ HT   ≈ SP

    ✕ Adh   ≋ Numb   ◯ rot   ╱ elev   � Short   ↔ Long

Documentation
for Wellness
Massage

Case Study: Lin Pak, a 38-year-old woman, is seeking monthly massage therapy for relaxation and stress reduction. She has type 1 diabetes and has been giving herself insulin injections 2 to 3 times per day since she was 12 years old. She has no health complications from her condition and wants to keep it that way. Her family has a history of heart disease, and she knows that diabetes further increases her chances of heart-related complications. She also knows that stress affects her blood-sugar levels. Lin is hoping massage therapy will provide her with new ways of handling the stress in her life and of keeping her heart strong and healthy.

Flow Charts: This flow chart demonstrates the forms that are recommended for use with clients seeking wellness care: who completes the form, how often the form is used, and any additional comments for using the form.

Wellness Care INTAKE FORMS	Who	Frequency	Comments
Fees and Policies	Client	Initial visit	Update as needed
Health Info—short version	Client	Initial visit	Update annually
Health Info—long version	—		
PROGRESS SUMMARIES			
Health Report	Client	Initial visit	Update every 6 to 8 tx
Progress Report	MT	Every 6 to 8 tx	Send to referring HCP
TREATMENT NOTES			
Wellness Chart	MT	Each visit	Record treatment; findings
Initial SOAP—long version	—		
Subsequent SOAP—short version	—		
Progress SOAP—long version	—		
Discharge SOAP—long version	—		
Range of Motion	—		

Naomi Wachtel

567 Sunnydale Dr.
Flat Irons, CO   80302
Tᴇʟ   303 555 8866

A. Fee Schedules

My Fees For Services Are As Follows:

Massage Therapy	$45 for 1/2 hour
97124	$80 for 1 hour

B. Payment Policies

Payment at time of service only.

C. Office Policies

Cancellations

Cancellations must be made 24 hours in advance of the scheduled appointment time. If cancellations are not made within 24 hours, payment in full is required. This charge will be waived if a replacement can be found for your appointment time. Your insurance company will not be charged for your missed appointment; you will be responsible for payment out-of-pocket.

Right of Refusal

I reserve the right to refuse service to anyone. This includes but is not limited to anyone who requests treatment or services that are outside my scope of practice. I will exercise this right if anyone arrives for treatment under the influence of alcohol or recreational drugs; I reserve the right to charge for the session time, whether or not services were rendered, if I so choose.

Patient Agreement

I have read the policies stated above and agree to abide by them.

Signature _Lin Pak_____   Date _7-27-04_____

Name _Lin Pak_   ID#/DOB _5-31-63_   Date _7-27-04_

Phone _(303) 555-0033x253_   Address _253 Boulder Rd., Flat Irons 80302_

1. What are your goals for health, and how may I assist you in achieving your goals? _Limit_
   longterm complications of diabetes through relaxation and stress reduction

2. List typical daily activities—work, exercise, home. _I sit a lot at work and watch movies_
   at home

3. Are you currently experiencing any of the following? If yes, please explain.

pain, tenderness	☒ No ☐ Yes: _____		stiffness	☒ No ☐ Yes: _____	
numbness or tingling	☒ No ☐ Yes: _____		swelling	☒ No ☐ Yes: _____	
allergies	☒ No ☐ Yes: _____				

4. List all illnesses, injuries, and health concerns you have now or have had in the past 3 years.
   (Examples: arthritis, diabetes, car crash, pregnancy) _diabetes, borderline high_
   blood pressure

5. List medications and pain relievers taken this week. _insulin_

6. I have provided all my known medical information. I acknowledge that massage therapy is
   not a substitute for medical diagnosis and treatment. I give my consent to receive treatment.

   Signature _Lin Pak_   Date _7-27-04_

   Tx: FB Sw Ⓝ, LDT neck, chest, axillary
        60 min.
   C: HW-relaxation ex., ✓ BP pre & post Ⓝ

Legend:

℮ TP	● TeP	○ Ⓟ	✳ Infl	≡ HT	≈ SP initials _NW, LMT_
✕ Adh	≋ Numb	↻ rot	╱ elev	⤜ Short	↔ Long

Naomi Wachtel
567 Sunnydale Dr.
Flat Irons, CO   80302
Tel   303 555 8866

HEALTH REPORT

Client Name ___Lin Pak___   Date ___7-27-04___

Date of Injury ___∅___   ID#/DOB ___5-31-63___

A. Draw today's symptoms on the figures.

1. Identify CURRENT symptomatic areas in your body by marking letters on the figures below.
   Use the letters provided in the key to identify the symptoms you are feeling today.
2. Circle the area around each letter, representing the size and shape of each symptom location.

Key
P = pain or tenderness
S = joint or muscle stiffness
N = numbness or tingling

B. Identify the intensity of your symptoms.

1. Pain Scale: Mark a line on the scale to show the amount of pain you are experiencing today.

   No Pain |———————————————————————————————| Unbearable Pain

2. Activities Scale: Mark a line on the scale to show the limitations you are experiencing today
   in your daily activities.

   Can Do Anything I Want |———————————————————————————————| Cannot Do Anything

C. Comments

   I get stiff in my chest, neck, and between my shoulder blades w/ long work days.

   Tx: FB Ⓜ SW & LDT to ↓ stiffness ↑ circ & ↑ relaxation

   M SH rot BL, HT chest, neck, midback L → L⁺, L Adh teres BL   NW, LMT

Signature ___Lin Pak___   Date ___7-27-04___

Naomi Wachtel
567 Sunnydale Dr.
Flat Irons, CO   80302
Tel   303 555 8866

WELLNESS CHART

Name _Lin Pak_____   ID#/DOB _5-31-63_   Meds _none_____

Tx: _FB SW Ⓜ, LDT_____
    _60 min_____
C: _HW con't_____

date _8-10-04_____   initials _NW, LMT_

Tx: _FB SW Ⓜ, LDT_____
    _60 min_____
C: _HW con't_____

date _8-24-04_____   initials _NW, LMT_

Tx: _FB SW Ⓜ, LDT_____
    _60 min_____
C: _pt rpt. BP ↓ post Ⓜ and overall_

date _9-7-04_____   initials _NW, LMT_

Tx: _FB SW Ⓜ, LDT_____
    _60 min_____
C: _flare-up worked overtime all wk_

date _9-21-04_____   initials _NW, LMT_

Legend:

℮ TP	• TeP	○ Ⓟ	⚹ Infl	≡ HT	≈ SP
✕ Adh	≋ Numb	⟲ rot	╱ elev	⊱ Short	⟷ Long

Naomi Wachtel
567 Sunnydale Dr.
Flat Irons, CO   80302
TEL   303 555 8866

Dr. Gregory Chandler
2323 Pill Hill
Flat Irons, CO 80309

Dear Dr. Chandler,

My client, Ms. Lin Pak, is a patient of yours. With her permission, I am writing to update you on her progress with massage therapy. Ms. Pak has been receiving bi-monthly massages for three months to promote relaxation and reduce the side effects of stress.

I have noted the following:
Posture—mild bilateral internal rotation of the shoulders and mild forward head position.
Tension—mild chest, neck and upper back.
Adhesions—mild shoulder.

I have used Swedish massage strokes and gentle lymphatic drainage to promote relaxation and enhance circulation and drainage. Ms. Pak has responded with a softening of her muscles, increased mobility in her shoulders, and her posture is returning to normal. Ms. Pak is doing breathing exercises at home which she finds very relaxing after a hard day at work. She tells me her blood pressure is lower for several days following her massages, which she'll be able to show you in her diary at her next appointment with you.

I will keep you informed of her progress with a short report every 6–8 sessions.

In health,
Naomi Wachtel

Documentation for Treatment Massage

Case Study: Darnel Washington, a 64-year-old retired male, sustained mild sprain-strain injuries typical of a motor vehicle collision, with moderate complications—the collision triggered the onset of previously dormant degenerative scoliosis. Mr. Washington was a passenger in a 1982 Honda Accord and was rear-ended by a 1991 Ford F250 truck. Mr. Washington was turned to the left talking with his nephew, the driver. They were driving to a hockey game, traffic was heavy, and road conditions were icy. He was wearing a seatbelt with a shoulder harness. They were slowing down to stop for a yellow light; the truck behind them was speeding up to go through the light. No ambulance was called to the scene. All involved drove away from the scene after assisting the police in filing a report. Mr. Washington and his nephew attended the remainder of the hockey game.

Initially, Mr. Washington felt fine, just a little stiff and sore. After a few weeks, his back pain worsened and headaches became more frequent. He scheduled an appointment with his physician who referred him to a massage therapist. Mr. Washington's massage therapist used manual lymphatic drainage, craniosacral therapy, and Feldenkrais as his primary treatment techniques.

Flow Charts: This flow chart demonstrates the forms that are recommended for use with clients with health concerns: who completes the form, how often the form is used, and any additional comments for using the form.

Treatment Massage	Who	Frequency	Comments
INTAKE FORMS			
Fees and Policies	Client	Initial visit	Update as needed
Health Info—short version	—		
Health Info—long version	Client	Initial visit	Update annually
PROGRESS SUMMARIES			
Health Report	Client	Monthly	Client reports current status
Progress Report	MT	Monthly	Practitioner reports to HCP
TREATMENT NOTES			
Wellness Chart	—		
Initial SOAP—long version	MT	Initial visit	Summarizes all findings; sets goals; creates treatment plan for next 30 days
Subsequent SOAP—short	MT	Each visit	(For use between initial, progress, and discharge sessions) brief; focus on treatment
Progress SOAP—long	MT	Monthly	Summarizes all findings; updates goals; updates treatment plan
Discharge SOAP—long	MT	Final visit	Summarizes all findings; status of functional progress; ongoing care plan
Range of Motion	MT	Monthly	Demonstrates pain and loss of movement; and ongoing progress toward normal, painfree movement

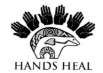

HANDS HEAL

John Olson, LMP, GCFP

345 Moon River Rd. Ste. 6
Minnehaha, MN   55987
Tel   612 555 9889

A. Fee Schedule

Fees for services are as follows:

• CranioSacral/Lymph Drainage (97140)	$100 per hour ($25 per 15 minute units)
• Feldenkrais (97112)	$100 per hour ($25 per 15 minute unit)
• Hot and Cold Packs (97010)	$15 per session ($15 per session)
• Therapeutic Massage (97124)	$80 Per Hour ($20 per 15 minute unit)

B. Payment Policies

Cash or Check

- A 10% discount is available when payment is made at the time services are provided.
- Pre-payment discounts: 6 sessions for the price of 5.

C. Office Policies

Cancellations

Cancellations must be made 24 hours in advance of the scheduled appointment time. If cancellations are not made within 24 hours, payment in full is required. This charge will be waived if a replacement can be found for your appointment time. Your insurance company will not be charged for your missed appointment; you will be responsible for payment out-of-pocket.

Right of Refusal

I reserve the right to refuse service to anyone. This includes but is not limited to anyone who requests treatment or services that are outside my scope of practice. I will exercise this right if anyone arrives for treatment under the influence of alcohol or recreational drugs; I reserve the right to charge for the session time, whether or not services were rendered, if I so choose.

Patient Agreement

I have read the policies stated above and agree to abide by them.

Signature   _Darnel G. Washington_____   Date   _2-6-01_____

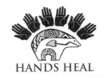

HANDS HEAL

John Olson, LMP, GCFP
345 Moon River Rd. Ste. 6
Minnehaha, MN   55987
TEL   612 555 9889

HEALTH INFORMATION

Client Name _Darnel G. Washington_   Date _2-6-04_

Date of Injury _1-6-04_   ID#/DOB _123-45-6789/4-22-37_

A. Client Information

Address _1209 Lake Winnetonka Dr._

City _Minnehaha_ State _MN_ Zip _55987_

Phone: Home _(612) 555-1515_

     Work _N/A_   Cell _555-5511_

Employer _IBM_

Work Address _N/A_

Occupation _retired_

Emergency Contact _Shalonda-wife_

Phone: Home _same_

     Work _N/A_   Cell _555-5511_

Primary Health Care Provider

Name _Sage Redtree, MD_

Address _87 Old Trail Pkwy_

City/State/Zip _Minnehaha MN 55987_

Phone: _555-0009_ Fax _555-9000_

I give my massage therapist permission to
consult with my health care providers
regarding my health and treatment.

Comments _____

Initials _DGW_   Date _2-6-02_

B. Current Health Information

List Health Concerns Check all that apply

Primary _back pain_
☐ mild ☒ moderate ☐ disabling
☒ constant ☐ intermittant
☐ symptoms ↑ w/activity   ☐ ↓ w/activity
☒ getting worse ☐ getting better ☐ no change
treatment received _pain pills, back brace_

Secondary _headaches_
☐ mild ☒ moderate ☐ disabling
☐ constant ☒ intermittant
☐ symptoms ↑ w/activity   ☐ ↓ w/activity
☒ getting worse ☐ getting better ☐ no change
treatment received _pain pills_

Additional _neck stiff_
☒ mild ☐ moderate ☐ disabling
☒ constant ☐ intermittant
☐ symptoms ↑ w/activity   ☐ ↓ w/activity
☐ getting worse ☒ getting better ☐ no change
treatment received _stretching_

List Daily Activities Limited by Condition

Work _N/A_

Home/Family _gardening, vacuuming_

Sleep/Self-care _sleep, exercise_

Social/Recreational _play w/ grandchildren,
dancing, bowling, bridge group_

List Self-Care Routines

How do you reduce stress? _watch sports,
garden_
Pain? _heat, back brace, meds_

List current medications (include pain relievers
and herbal remedies) _____
hydrocodone 500 mg every 4 hrs

_____

Have you ever received massage therapy
before? _no_   Frequency? _____

What are your goals for receiving massage
therapy? _get around easier, less pain_

_____

C. Health History

List and Explain. Include dates and treatment
received.

Surgeries _appendicitis 1949 removed,
torn meniseus ⊙ knee 1980 arthoscopy_

_____

Injuries _bowling injury ⊙ knee 1979
no treatment until surgery 1980_

_____

Major Illnesses _scoliosis 1949
Milwaukee brace, exercise, pain meds_

160

Check All Current and Previous Conditions   Please Explain

General

current	past		comments
☒	☐	headaches	_____
☒	☒	pain _scoliosis_	
☒	☐	sleep disturbances	
		can't get comfortable	
☐	☒	fatigue _scoliosis_	
☐	☐	infections	_____
☐	☐	fever	_____
☐	☐	sinus	_____
☐	☐	other	_____

Skin Conditions

current	past		comments
☐	☐	rashes	_____
☐	☐	athlete's foot, warts	____
☐	☐	other	_____

Muscles and Joints

current	past		comments
☐	☐	rheumatoid arthritis	
☒	☐	osteoarthritis	_____
☐	☐	osteoporosis	_____
☒	☒	scoliosis	_____
☐	☐	broken bones	_____
☐	☐	spinal problems	_____
☐	☐	disk problems	_____
☐	☐	lupus	_____
☐	☐	TMJ, jaw pain	_____
☐	☐	spasms, cramps	
☐	☐	sprains, strains	
☐	☐	tendonitis, bursitis	
☐	☐	stiff or painful joints	____
☐	☒	weak or sore muscles	
		scoliosis	
☐	☐	neck, shoulder, arm pain	
☒	☒	low back, hip, leg pain	
		MVA, scoliosis	
☐	☐	other	_____

Nervous System

current	past		comments
☐	☐	head injuries, concussions	
☐	☐	dizziness, ringing in ears	
☐	☐	loss of memory, confusion	
☐	☐	numbness, tingling	
☐	☐	sciatica, shooting pain	
☐	☐	chronic pain	_____
☐	☐	depression	_____
☐	☐	other	_____

Respiratory, Cardiovascular

current	past		comments
☐	☐	heart disease	_____
☐	☐	blood clots	_____
☐	☐	stroke	_____
☐	☐	lymphadema	_____
☐	☐	high, low blood pressure	
☐	☐	irregular heart beat	
☐	☐	poor circulation	_____
☐	☐	swollen ankles	_____
☐	☐	varicose veins	_____
☐	☐	chest pain, shortness of breath	_____
☐	☐	asthma	_____

Allergies

current	past		comments
☐	☐	scents, oils, lotions	____
☐	☐	detergents	_____
☐	☐	other	_____

Digestive/Elimination System

current	past		comments
☐	☐	bowel problems	_____
☐	☐	gas, bloating	_____
☐	☐	bladder/kidney/prostrate	
☐	☐	abdominal pain	_____
☐	☐	other	_____

Endocrine System

current	past		comments
☐	☐	thyroid	_____
☐	☐	diabetes	_____

Reproductive System

current	past		comments
☐	☐	pregnancy	_____
☐	☐	painful, emotional menses	
☐	☐	fibrotic cysts	_____

Cancer/Tumors

current	past		comments
☐	☐	benign	_____
☐	☐	malignant	_____

Habits

current	past		comments
☐	☒	tobacco	_quit chew 30 yrs ago_
☐	☐	alcohol	_____
☐	☐	drugs	_____
☒	☐	coffee, soda	_1-2 cups/day_

Contract for Care

I promise to participate fully as a member of my health care team. I will make sound choices regarding my treatment plan based on the information provided by my massage therapist and other members of my health care team, and my experience of those suggestions. I agree to participate in the self care program we select. I promise to inform my practitioner any time I feel my well-being is threatened or compromised. I expect my massage therapist to provide safe and effective treatment.

Consent for Care

It is my choice to receive massage therapy, and I give my consent to receive treatment. I have reported all health conditions that I am aware of and will inform my practitioner of any changes in my health.

Signature _Darnel G. Washington_   Date _2-6-04_

HANDS HEAL

John Olson, LMP, GCFP
345 Moon River Rd. Ste. 6
Minnehaha, MN   55987
TEL   612 555 9889

HEALTH REPORT

Client Name ___Darnel G. Washington_____   Date _2-6-04_____

Date of Injury __1-6-04_____   ID#/DOB _123-45-6789/4-22-37_____

A. Draw today's symptoms on the figures.

1. Identify CURRENT symptomatic areas in your body by marking letters on the figures below.
   Use the letters provided in the key to identify the symptoms you are feeling today.
2. Circle the area around each letter, representing the size and shape of each symptom location.

Key
P = pain or tenderness
S = joint or muscle stiffness
N = numbness or tingling

B. Identify the intensity of your symptoms.

1. Pain Scale: Mark a line on the scale to show the amount of pain you are experiencing today.

   No Pain |————————————•————————————| Unbearable Pain   (5.5)

2. Activities Scale: Mark a line on the scale to show the limitations you are experiencing today
   in your daily activities.   (5.5)

   Can Do Anything I Want |————————————•————————————| Cannot Do Anything

C. Comments

_____
_____
_____
_____

Signature __Darnel G. Washington_____   Date _2-6-04_____

![Hands Heal logo]()

John Olson, LMP, GCFP
345 Moon River Rd. Ste. 6
Minnehaha, MN   55987
TEL   612 555 9889

HANDS HEAL

SOAP CHART-M

Client Name ___Darnel G. Washington___   Date _2-6-04_

Date of Injury ___1-6-04___   ID#/DOB _123-45-6789_ Meds ___hydrocodone 500 mg q4h___

S   Focus Health Concerns: Prioritize   ↓ ⓟ hd, C, T, L

   Symptoms: Location/Intensity/Frequency/Duration/Onset

   C, T, L ⓟ M Con post MVC   Δ L

   HA ⓟ M interm/da post MVC   Δ ⓟ

   Activities of Daily Living: Aggravating/Relieving
   1. lift GD c̄ M+ ⓟ = carseat, highchair, crib
   2. gardening s ⓟ p̄ 5 min = veg & flowers, time c̄ wife
   3. unable to sit & play bridge after 30 min.
   R: rest, heat

O   Findings: Visual/Palpable/Test Results
   V: 1° WB rising and standing - Ⓡ leg & Ft L Δ bal
      sits Ⓡ pelvis, bends mid - T Ⱥ
      BR M shallow RR Δ L & even
      L-M seg mvm't Ⓛ ribs c̄ deep inh Δ smooth
   P: M Ⓡ frontal tor Δ L
      M+ Ⓑⓛ sph decomp Δ M
      L+ Adh tent Ⱥ
      CSR M weak Ⓡ L Ⓛ
         Δ L   Δ N

   Techniques/Modalities: Locations/Duration

   97140   LDT trunk   Fl eyes & ft
   60 min.   CST hd

   Response to Treatment (see Δ)

A   Goals: Long-term/Short-term
   LTG: Lift GD 10x/da from floor to carry
   10 min 5 da/wk c̄ L ⓟ & fatigue-60 da
   STG: Lift light weight toys from floor 10x/da
   3 da/wk c̄ L ⓟ -2 wks

   Functional Outcomes

P   Future Treatment/Frequency
   2x/wk for 3 wks, 60 min/tx
   LDT, CST, Fl-ribs, diap., ↑ mob ↓ Adh

   Homework/Self-care
   con't heat T, ice only C, L
   Deep BR ex

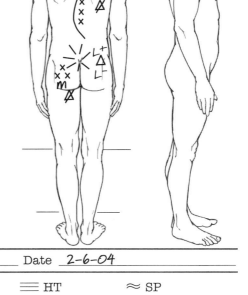

Therapist's Signature ___JO, LMP, GCFP___   Date _2-6-04_

Legend:
ⓔ TP	• TeP	○ ⓟ	⚹ Infl	≡ HT	≈ SP
✕ Adh	≷ Numb	↺ rot	╱ elev	⊶ Short	↔ Long

John Olson, LMP, GCFP
345 Moon River Rd. Ste. 6
Minnehaha, MN   55987
TEL   612 555 9889

HANDS HEAL

SOAP CHART-M

Client Name ___Darnel G. Washington___   Date __2-8-04__

Date of Injury __1-6-04__   ID#/DOB __123-45-6789__ Meds __hydrocodone 500 mg q4h__

S Focus-decrease pain in head and neck

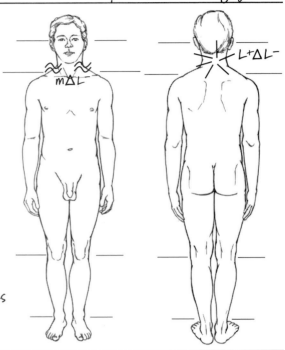

O 97140   60 min
    Lymph Drainage neck, head

A F.O.-lifting lightweight toys from shelves with
    moderate pain

P having good success with ice and breathing exercises
    con't as instructed

Therapist's Signature ___JO LMP GCFP___   Date ___2-8-04___

S Focus-decrease pain in head & neck

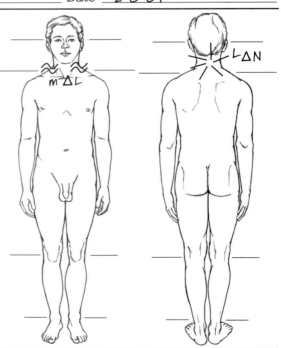

O 97140 60 min
    Lymph Drainage neck, head, chest, arms,
    all passive cervical ranges of motion limited-mild
    minus-with mild pain at end ranges Δ N
    with L⁻ pain
A con't

P con't

Therapist's Signature ___JO LMP GCFP___   Date ___2-11-04___

Legend: ℮ TP   • TeP   ○ Ⓟ   ✳ Infl   ≡ HT   ≈ SP
         ✕ Adh   ≷ Numb   ◯ rot   ╱ elev   ⊱ Short   ↔ Long

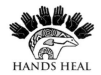

HANDS HEAL

John Olson, LMP, GCFP

345 Moon River Rd. Ste. 6
Minnehaha, MN   55987
TEL   612 555 9889

Dr. Sage Redtree
87 Old Trail Parkway
Minnehaha, MN 55987

Client: Darnel G. Washington
DOI: 1-6-01
Insurance ID #: 123-45-6789

3-8-04

Dear Dr. Redtree:

Thank you for the referral of Mr. Washington. We have had six treatments in the last 30 days. In this time he has reached his initial short-term goal of being able to lift lightweight toys from the floor up to a high shelf at least 10 times a day, three days a week—on the days that he takes care of his granddaughter—with no more than mild pain in his back. We have also resolved the inflammation in his neck and reduced his headaches to mild and infrequent.

Mr. Washington has yet to accomplish his long-term goal of lifting his granddaughter at least 10 times a day and carrying her at least 10 minutes twice a day during the three days a week he cares for her. To support him in accomplishing this goal, I would like to continue to see Mr. Washington twice per week for one hour sessions of Manual Lymphatic Drainage, CranioSacral Therapy, and Feldenkrais. My goals are to reduce the scar tissue and muscle spasms in his neck and back and improve the mobility of his ribs, neck, and shoulders. Mr. Washington will continue to use alternating heat and ice packs on his neck and back as per the handouts and instructions I have provided, and he is diligent about doing the breathing exercises as instructed.

Please let me know by fax if this treatment plan is acceptable to you.

I am aware that Mr. Washington has a history of scoliosis, and I have asked him to schedule an appointment with you for an evaluation of that condition. I am concerned that it may interfer with his progress.

Sincerely,
John Olson, LMP, GCFP

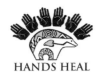

John Olson, LMP, GCFP
345 Moon River Rd. Ste. 6
Minnehaha, MN   55987
TEL   612 555 9889

HANDS HEAL

SOAP CHART—M

Client Name _Darnel G. Washington_   Date _1-20-04_

Date of Injury _1-6-04_   ID#/DOB _123-45-6789_ Meds _Ø_

S Focus for Today   ↓ stiff back

Symptoms: Location/Intensity/Frequency/Duration/Onset
Stiff T L cons, 4 da-bridge marathon 2-7—05
Δ WNL

Activities of Daily Living: Aggravating/Relieving
A: carrying GD ↑ 10 min, sit or garden ↑ 2 hrs = ↑ Ⓟ M
R: ex, stretch, rest

O Findings: Visual/Palpable/Test Results
M weak c̄ sit Δ L
mvm't T vs hip
rib mob M ↓   BR L ↓ Δ N
Δ L

Techniques/Modalities: Locations/Duration
97140   Fl ribs T
60 min   CST — C, T, L trac c̄ unwinding
Response to Treatment (see Δ)

A Goals: Long-term/Short-term
all goals have been reached within the limits of
current health condition

Functional Outcomes
has not regained prior functional status since
MVA 1-6-04 (see ADLS)

P Future Treatment/Frequency
con't ATM classes 1x/wk, ↑ prn
released from care, ref. to P̄ HCP

Homework/Self-care
BR ex ribroll ex c̄ ↑ sit
rest + ex ā stiff

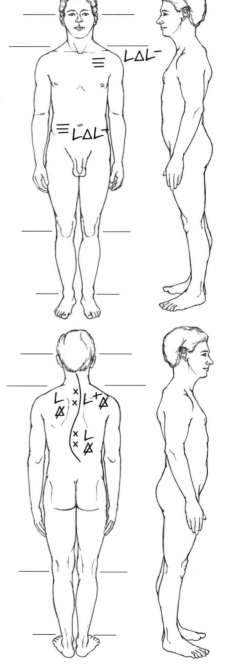

Therapist's Signature _JO LMP, GCFP_   Date _1-20-04_

Legend: ℮ TP   • TeP   ○ Ⓟ   ✳ Infl   ≡ HT   ≈ SP
              ✕ Adh   ≋ Numb   ◯ rot   ╱ elev   ⤙ Short   ↔ Long

166   Copyright © 2005 Lippincott Williams & Wilkins

Appendix C
Abbreviations List

HANDS HEAL ESSENTIALS:
DOCUMENTATION
FOR MASSAGE THERAPISTS

Symbols

ā, pre	before
@	at
&, +	and
~ , ˜	approximate
c̄, w/	with
D	change
↓	down, decrease
=	equals
♀	female
>	greater than
→	leading to, resulting in, through
♂	male
–	minus, negative
#	number
Ø	no, none
p̄, post	after
//	parallel
/	per
1°	primary
+	plus, positive
s̄, w/o	without
2°	secondary, because of
x	times, repetitions
↑	up, increase

Symbols for figure drawing:

✕	adhesion
╱	elevation
≡	hypertonicity, tension
↔	longer than normal
≳	numbness, tingling
Ⓟ	pain
↻	rotation
⟩⟨	shorter than normal
≈	spasm
✳	swelling, inflammation
●	tender points
ⓔ	trigger point

Anatomy: (Sample list of common landmarks. Follow suit with additional terms by shortening words or using initials.)

abs	abdominals
AC	acromioclavicular
ACL	anterior crutiate ligament
AIIS	anterior inferior iliac spine
ASIS	anterior superior iliac spine
ATFL	anterior talofibular ligament
AW	abdominal wall
BBB	blood brain barrier
BEF	bioenergetic field
bi	biceps
BJM	bones, joints, and muscles
BR	breath
C, C 1-7	cervical, cervical vertebrae
CN 1-8	cervical nerves
CrN 1-12	cranial nerves
CSF	cerebral spinal fluid
ch	chest
Cl	clavicle
CM	carpometacarpal
CNS	central nervous system
coc	coccygeal
Cr	cranium
delt	deltoid
DH	dominant hand
dia	diaphragm
E	energy
elb	elbow
EMF	electromagnetic field
ES	erector spinae muscle group
FE	femur
gastroc	gastrocnemius
GHL	glenohumeral ligament
gluts	gluteal muscle group
GT	greater trochanter
hams	hamstring muscles
he	heart
hd	head
H&N	head and neck
hum	humerus
IC	ileocecal, iliococcygeal, intercarpal, intercostal, intracranial
IF	iliofemoral
IP	iliopsoas
ISF	interstitial fluid
ITB	iliotibial band
IT	ischial tuberosity
IVD	intervertebral disk
IVJC	intervertebral joint complex
J, jt	joint
JV	jugular vein
L, L 1-5	lumbar, lumbar vertebrae
LC	lymph capillaries
LCL	lateral collateral ligament
lats	latissimus dorsi
lev scap	levator scapulae
LI	large intestine
LN	lymph node
LV	lymph vessel
mas	masseter
meta	metacarpal, metatarsal
mm	muscles
MN	median nerve
ms	musculoskeletal
nn	nerves
NR	nerve root
NS	nervous system
occ	occiput
OF	occipitofrontal
os	bone
PCx	paracervical
pecs; M&m	pectoralis major and minor
PNS	parasympathetic nervous system
PSIS	posterior sacroiliac spine, posterior superior iliac spine
Q	radiant energy
QL	quadratus lumborum
quads	quadricep muscles
RC	rib cage
rhomb	rhomboids
SB	sternal border
SC	subclavian, sternoclavicular, sternocostal
sc	subcutaneous
SCM	sternocleidomastoid
ScM	scalene muscle group
SCV	subclavian vein
SI	sacroiliac, small intestine
sh	shoulder
sol	soleus
ST	soft tissue
st	sternum
T, T 1-12	thoracic, thoracic vertebrae
TC	thoracic cage
TD	thoracic duct
TFA	tibiofemoral angle
TFL	tensor fascia lata
th	throat
tib	tibia, tibialis
tibfib	tibia and fibula
TMJ	temporomandibular joint
traps	trapezius
tri	triceps
UN	ulnar nerve
vert	vertebrae
visc	viscera

Descriptive Terms:

Abn	abnormal
aux	auxiliary
avg	average
cons	constant
F	fair
freq	frequent
G	good
G&B	good and bad (days)
grad	gradual
interm	intermittent
L	light, low, mild
Ltd	limited, limitation
M	moderate
max	maximum
min	minimum
N	normal
OK	all right, acceptable
P	poor
QOL	quality of life
QWL	quality of working life
rig	rigid
S	severe
seg	segmented
seld	seldom
sm	smooth
Sp	spastic
sym	symmetrical
VGH	very good health
WNL	within normal limits
xs	excessive

Directions and Positions

adj	adjacent, adjoining, adjuctive
ant	anterior,
Ⓑ, ⒝ⓛ	bilateral, both
cd	caudal
ceph	cephalic
D/3	distal third
dist	distal
dp	deep
ext	external
glob	global
inf	inferior
int	internal
inter	between
intra	within
Ⓛ	left
L/3	lower third
lat	lateral
LE	lower extremities
LQ	lower quadrant
M/3	middle third
med	medial
ML	midline

OL — other location
P/3 — proximal third
post — posterior
prox — proximal
pr — prone
Ⓡ — right
SL — sidelying
sup — superior, supine
super — superficial
U/3 — upper third
UE — upper extremities
unilat — unilateral
univ — universal
UQ — upper quadrant

Movements and Planes of Movement

abd — abduction
act — activities
add — adduction
ADLs — activities of daily living
art — articulate
circ — circumduction
dep — depression
DF — dorsiflexion
ele — elevation
ever — eversion
ext — external
flex — flexion
FM — functional movement
front — frontal
inv — inversion
lat flex — lateral flexion
mob — mobility
mvmt — movement
opp — opposition
PF — plantarflexion
pro — pronation
Ptx — protraction
ROM — range of motion
  AROM — active range of motion
  AAROM — active assisted range of motion
  PROM — passive range of motion
  RROM — resistive range of motion
  CPROM — complete and pain-free range of motion
rot — rotation
Rtx — retraction
sag — sagittal
SB — sidebending
sh — shear
sup — supination
tor — torsion
trans — transverse

Measurements and Medical Record Terminology

A: — assessment
a.c. — before meals
ACI — after-care instructions
am — morning
AMAP — as much as possible
a.p. — before dinner
appt — appointment
ASAP — as soon as possible
b.i.d. — twice a day
bpm — beats per minute
cm — centimeter
CNT — could not test
c/o — complains of
COD — condition on discharge
cont — continue
cpm — counts or cycles per minute
CSR — craniosacral rhythm
CSTx — continue same treatment
D — daughter
da — day
D/C — discharged or discontinued
DD — daily
DKA — did not keep appointment
DNT — did not test
DOB — date of birth
DOI — date of injury
dur — duration
ea — each
EOD — every other day
FB — full body
freq — frequency
ft — foot
GD — granddaughter
GF — grandfather
GM — grandmother
gm — gram
GS — grandson
h.d., h.s. — at bedtime
hr — hour
hgt — height
h.v. — this evening
Hx — history
i.c. — between meals
ID — identification
immed — immediately
in — inches
int — intensity
kg — kilogram
kph — kilometers per hour
l — liter
lb — pound
lpm — liter per minute
LTG — long-term goal

M — mother
m.d., m.g. — as directed
meds — medications
mg — milligrams
min — minutes
ml — milliliters
mm — millimeters
mo — month
mph — mile per hour
nv — next visit
O: — objective
ODAT — one day at a time
o.h., q.h. — every hour
o.m., q.m. — every morning
o.n., q.n. — every night
ons — onset
oz — ounce
P: — plan
p.c., p.p. — after meals
pg — page
pls — please
pm — afternoon, evening
POMR — Problem-Oriented Medical Record
ppm — pulses per minute
prn — as needed
PTD — prior to discharge
q2h — every two hours
q3h — every three hours
q.i.d — four times daily
q.l. — as much as desired
q.o.d — every other day
reps — repetitions
RR — respiratory rate
Rx — drugs, prescription, medication, therapy
S — son
S: — subjective
S/A — same as
SAA — same as above
SATx — same treatment
sched — schedule
sec — seconds
s.i.d., u.i.d — once a day
SOAP — Subjective, Objective, Assessment, Plan
stat — at once
STG — short-term goal
suc — success
t.d.d., t.i.d. — three times a day
t.i.w. — three times a week
TMTC — too many to count
TST — total sleep time
UFN — until further notice
unk — unknown

Symptoms and Maladies

Abr — abrasion
Acc — accident

Adh — adhesion
AE — acute exacerbation
AI — accidental injury
AIDS — autoimmune deficiency syndrome
ANI — acute nerve irritation
AOB — alcohol on breath
ASP — abnormal spine posture
atr — atrophy
BA — back ache
CA — cancer
CFS — chronic fatigue syndrome
CHD — coronary heart disease
CHI — closed head injury
CHS — congestive heart failure
CHT — closed head trauma
CP — cerebral palsy
crep — crepitis
CTS — carpal tunnel syndrome
DDD — degenerative disk disease
DJD — degenerative joint disease
Dx — diagnosis
EC — energy cyst
ed — edema
EM — emotional, early memory
FB — foreign body
flac — flaccid
FLR — funny looking rash
Flat — flatulence
Fl up — flare up
FOOSH — fell on outstretched hand
FM, FMS — fibromyalgia
FT — fibrous tissue
HA — headache
HD — heart disease, herniated disk
HI — head injury
HNP — herniated nucleus pulposus
Hnt — hypertension
HOH — hard of hearing
HT — hypertonicity, tension, tight muscles
HTR — hypertrophy
Infl — inflammation
AI — acute inflammation, phase I

SI	subacute inflammation, phase II
CI	chronic inflammation, phase III
JRA	juvenile rheumatoid arthritis
kyph	kyphosis
lax	laxity
LB	loose bodies
LD	learning disability
les	lesion
LJM	limited joint mobility
LOC	loss of consciousness
LOM	loss of movement
lord	lordosis
MAEW	moves all extremities well
MI	myocardial infarction
MPS	myofascial pain syndrome
NRI	nerve root irritation
NSI	no sign of infection, inflammation
OA	osteoarthritis
Ⓟ	pain
para	paraplegia
PCS	postconcussive syndrome
PD	perception disorder
PNP	peripheral neuropathy
POM	pain on motion
PTSD	posttraumatic stress disorder
Px	prognosis
RA	rheumatoid arthritis
RSS	repetitive stress syndrome
RTD	repetitive trauma disorder
SCI	spinal cord injury
SD	sleep disturbances
SFLE	stress from life experience
SL	subluxation
SOB	shortness of breath
SOBOE	shortness of breath on exercise
Sp	spasm, spastic
st	stiffness

STS	soft tissue swelling
STI	soft tissue injury
Sw	swelling
Sx	symptoms
TBI	traumatic brain injury
TeP	tender point
TJA	total joint arthrotomy or arthroplasty
THA	total hip arthrotomy or arthroplasty
TKA	total knee arthrotomy or arthroplasty
TJR	total joint replacement
TAR	total ankle replacement
TER	total elbow replacement
THR	total hip replacement
TKR	total knee replacement
TSR	total shoulder replacement
TOS	thoracic outlet syndrome
TP	trigger point
URI	upper respiratory infection
UTI	urinary tract infection
VGH	very good health
VV	vericose vein

Treatments, Modalities, Findings

AAS	active assisted stretching
AC	acupuncture, acupressure
AKS	arthroscopic knee surgery
aroma	aromatherapy
AT	adjunctive therapy
bal	balance
B&B	bowel and bladder function
BM	bowel movement
BJE	bone and joint exam
BP	blood pressure
BRS	breath sounds
BV	steam bath
C&E	consultation and examination
chak	chakra

contra	contraindicated
coord	coordinate
CP	cold packs
CST	craniosacral therapy
DB	deep breathing
DBE	deep breathing exercise
detox	detoxification
DP	direct pressure
DT	deep tissue
eff	effleurage
erg	ergonomics consultation
EW	energy work
Ex	exercise
exam	examination
FS	facilitated stretching
FWB	full weight-bearing
Fx	friction
HARPPS	signs of infection: heat, absence of use, redness, pain, pus, swelling
H&C	hot and cold
HEP	home exercise program
HMP	hot moist packs
HP	hot packs
HW	homework
hydro	hydrotherapy
ICES	ice, compression, elevation, support
IDM	indirect method
immob	immobilize
JM	joint mobility
jos	jostling
LAM	laminectomy
LAP	laproscopy
LBPQ	low back pain questionnaire
LDT	lymphatic drainage technique
LT	light touch
Ⓜ	massage
man	manipulation
mer	meridian
MET	muscle energy technique
MFT	muscle function test
MFR	myofascial release
MH	moist heat
MLD	manual lymphatic drainage
MT	manual therapy
NA	not attempted
N/A	not applicable
NMT	neuromuscular therapy
NP	not palpable

NWB	non-weight-bearing
OBE	out-of-body experience
obs	observation
O&E	observation and examination
OE	orthopedic examination
os adj	osseous adjustment
OTB	off the body
PA	postural analysis or assessment
palp	palpation
PB	parafin bath, postural balancing
pet	petrissage
PMP	pain management program
PNF	proprioceptive neuromuscular facilitation
PPR	passive positional release
PR	postural re-education
PRE	progressive resistive exercise
prev	prevention
proc	procedure
PT	physical therapy
PU	props utilized
PVD	percussion, vibration, drainage
PWB	partial weight-bearing
R&E	rest and exercise
re-ed	re-education
reflex	reflexology
re-x	re-examination
ROS	review of symptoms, review of systems
RR	respiratory rate
RT	recreational therapy
RTW	return to work
SA	skeletal alignment
SAE	specific action exercise
SC	self-care
SDTx	sleeps during treatment
SE	somatic education
SER	somato-emotional release
SET	subtle energy techniques
SLR	straight leg raise
S&S	stretching and strengthening
str	stretching

SU	supports utilized	tx	traction	VAPS	visual analog pain scale
TENS	transcutaneous electrical nerve stimulation	Ptx	pelvic traction	VS	vascular flush
		Ltx	lumbar traction	WB	weight-bearing
Tx	treatment	Ttx	thoracic traction	XFF	cross fiber friction
		Ctx	cervical traction		

Index

Page numbers in *italics* indicate figures. *Blank Forms* are designated as such.